RIC

THE GUY'S GUIDE
to Everything
BREAST CANCER

foreword by
DOUGLAS HOWE

Chapter Contributors:
DR. CARLA GARCIA
MR. KHEVIN BARNES

BBF Publishing & *Enterprises*

The Guy's Guide To Everything Breast Cancer
Copyright © 2021 by Rick Baker. All rights reserved.

No part of this publication may be reproduced, stored in a retrieval system or transmitted in any way by any means, electronic, mechanical, photocopy, recording or otherwise without the prior permission of the author except as provided by USA copyright law.

The opinions expressed by the author are not necessarily those of BBF Publishing CO.

Published by BBF Publishing & Enterprises
POB 62130 | Colorado Springs, CO 80920 USA
1.719.822.2328 | www.beckybakerfdn.org

BBF Publishing is committed to excellence in the publishing industry. The company is the publishing arm of The Becky Baker Foundation, a 501(C)(3) nonprofit charity committed to preventing breast cancer.

Book design copyright © 2021 by BBF Publishing CO. All rights reserved.
Cover design by Mohsin Sheikh
Interior design by Kristin Waller

Published in the United States of America

ISBN: 978-0-578-86026-8
1. Women's Health
2. Cancer, Breast
11.01.10

Printed in the United States of America
Signature Book Printing, www.sbpbooks.com

Foreword

What would you do if you inherited a million dollars, today?! Or, what would you do if you hit the lottery for a million dollars? What would you do with the money?

Rick Baker is a talented friend and the founder of the Becky Baker Foundation, and the million-dollar scenario emerged for him when, after going through the painful final years of his wife's life, he received a one-million-dollar life insurance check.

To honor Becky, he used the funds to launch the Becky Baker Foundation, providing mammograms and thermograms to assist women in the most important step of cancer prevention, which is early detection and identification.

Yes, you read that right. Rick didn't spend it on a mansion of a home, or worldwide travel, or man toys. He invested in tangible cancer prevention steps for women, launching a nationwide movement to detect breast cancer at the earliest possible stage and spare countless women from the pain and eventual premature end of Becky Baker's life.

Education on this matter is important; getting a mammogram or thermogram is even more important, and that is what the Foundation provides.

I have the privilege of serving on the Board of the Becky Baker Foundation, playing a small role in our big quest to help as many women as possible with the kind of early detection that is most necessary to preventing breast cancer. And in this, the latest in the line of Rick Baker's purpose-driven books, Rick shares with all of us men (and women, too!) what we need to know about breast cancer, and how we can take potentially life-saving steps to help protect the vibrant lives of our wives, moms, adult daughters, and friends.

You may not have won the million dollars, but in these pages you'll get to learn from the guy who did.

I've had the opportunities of writing two short books, blogging for FoxFaith and authoring a weekly inspirational letter to men, so I recognize good writing skill in others and Rick has it.

As a professional business consultant and Executive Coach, I know that good leaders need good information to make good decisions. Herein lies a smart book that skillfully gives us good information so that we can make good decisions (or at least offer them) to those ladies we love. And, in Chapter Four, you'll learn about how men can get breast cancer, too.

Most of us don't sit together at the club or the Pub or the coffee house discussing cancer. And when men are talking about breasts its usually in the context of sexual objects and not ticking time bombs.

Rick starts there and launches into the kind of knowledge we could all use, moving from breasts to cancer to the cure to care to continuity.

I commend it to you and may women you know – and especially women you love – be the beneficiaries, living out their days with high hopes, long-lasting dreams, and lots of years ahead to achieve and enjoy the plethora of opportunities that await them before their time on earth is done.

Rev. Doug Howe
Director, Insignia Foundation

Table of Contents

Preface

Section One: Understanding This Evil Disease

Chapter 1: Sexual Objects, or Ticking Timebombs?
Chapter 2: A Practical Definition of "The Breast"
Chapter 3: How Does It Start and Where Does It Come From?
Chapter 4: Men Get Breast Cancer Too?
Chapter 5: The Man and The Mammogram
Chapter 6: Will There Ever Be a Cure?
Chapter 7: What About This Pink Ribbon?
Chapter 8: The Prostitution of The Pink Ribbon

Section Two: Preventing Breast Cancer in Your Loved One

Chapter 9:   Supporting Your Loved One At All Costs
Chapter 10: Becky's LAFF2LIVE Program
Chapter 11: Designing Your Own Proactive Plan
Chapter 12: Knowing Breast Cancer Stages
Chapter 13: The Oncologist Plays God

Epilogue: Never Give Up

Preface

On December 17, 2013, my wife Becky and I, were shopping at COSTCO when she stubbed her toe on our grocery cart and fell to the ground screaming in pain. She told me to take her to the Emergency Room immediately. I didn't understand her panic, as all she did was stub her toe. But, off to Wake Forest Baptist Hospital we went.

Once there, Becky was assigned a bed in the Emergency Room, complete with those white curtains that slide for privacy. Tests were run, Becky was poked and prodded, and after two hours, she was to be transferred to a hospital room suite on the top floor of the hospital.

Becky seemed to know why, but I sure didn't. All she did was stub her toe. I wondered what I was missing?

We headed up the elevator to the "penthouse" area of the hospital. The elevator stopped, the doors opened, and there it was: a large sign that read, "Comprehensive Cancer Center." *Cancer Center?* All she did was stub her toe!

Becky was lovingly escorted to her suite as I followed behind, now in a daze. She was helped into the large bed, near the full-length picture window that overlooked all of Winston-Salem, North Carolina.

The head oncologist arrived and chatted with Becky, then asked me to follow her out of the suite and into the hallway as Becky was getting into bed.

With not an ounce of compassion or warmth, she blurted out, almost like a robot, these words:

"Becky has stage IV metastatic ER Positive Breast Cancer. She has three months to live, so get your affairs in order."

It was as if someone had just punched me in the stomach. I said, "How can this be? All she did was stub her toe."

"No," said the oncologist. "Becky has had breast cancer for over a year; she has just hidden it from you and everyone else, until she couldn't any longer. When she stubbed her toe at COSTCO, she actually fractured two more ribs, as her bones are now like eggshells."

I recount for you Becky's story for one reason and one reason alone: I don't want *our* story to ever become *your* story.

Back then, breast cancer was nothing more to me than a pink ribbon on an NFL football in October. I was clueless. Breasts, to me, were sexual objects to be enjoyed. I had no idea they could be ticking timebombs.

I have written this book so that you and your wife, girlfriend, mother, or other loved one, will not be faced with what Becky and I were.

You will read that Becky did not die in three months — as the arrogant doctors told her she would. But against all odds, she lived 37 months beyond those three, and in her passing, she has saved hundreds of women from this disease. It is my prayer that this book will save your loved one (and you) from this life-altering monster of a disease.

Breast cancer *is* preventable in many women. While your loved one may not have this evil disease today, remember that close to one-in-seven women in the U.S. will be diagnosed with breast cancer in their lifetime. It is an epidemic.

Before Becky stubbed her toe that fateful day at COSTCO, our lives together were a fairy tale. Then suddenly everything changed, and nothing would ever be the same again.

I like to say that 'Becky's not gone, she's just not here.' I believe with all my heart, that if she could, she would encourage you — as a guy — to become an expert in understanding this evil disease so that you will be equipped to help your loved one prevent it, for the rest of your lives.

Rick Baker

Section One

Understanding This Evil Disease

Chapter One
Sexual Objects, or Ticking Timebombs?

*"The greatest enemy of knowledge is not ignorance,
it is the illusion of knowledge."*
— **Daniel J. Boorstin**

If you are like I was back in 2013 when Becky was first diagnosed with breast cancer, you probably don't have a clear picture of what this disease is, how or why women get it, or if it is preventable.

Let's talk like guys, shall we? We love breasts. Many men are addicted to breasts. Hollywood knows this and displays them at every turn. If they are not allowed to show the complete breast, they tease men with erotic clothing designed to pique our interest, which seems to fascinate many Europeans.

Across the Big Pond, women go topless at beaches and in public as a common occurrence. Not so in America. The American male almost worships women's breasts that remain hidden from view (mostly) in public.

I am reminded of a morning years ago, when I was a pastor in Austin, Texas. I was sitting in my car, stopped at a red light on Sixth Street in downtown, headed to my favorite breakfast joint, when a female jogger approached the intersection. The light was green for her, so she continued to jog through the intersection right past the hood of my car. As she passed me, she turned and smiled, and as I looked at her, my eyes did not believe what they saw. She was *topless*. Yep, jogging through that intersection with her breasts free as the breeze! Here I was, a senior pastor for a large congregation, and I still stared. Not sinfully, mind you, but in admiration. (Sheepish smile)

I was not the only guy in the area, and horns started blaring as the signal had turned green with all guys frozen in place.

Breasts, for most American men, are sexual objects. We love our wife's breasts, and she probably loves that you love them. They are a vital part of our intimacy with our spouse or girlfriend, and they know this, which can cause a serious problem in our relationship. How so?

Let's back up a bit. What I did not mention in my preface was that Becky had found a lump the size of a BB in her left breast nine months before she was diagnosed with stage IV breast cancer.

She didn't tell anyone. Not me, her family, her friends, or her doctor. I would find out about the small lump from her mother, just a few months before Becky would pass away. She had finally told her mom about what she had found and how she was afraid to get a mammogram because of what it would mean. In fact, Becky had never had a mammogram. Not in 53 years. (She was not alone as most studies seem to indicate that half the women in America have never had a breast cancer screening.)

When I talked to Becky about this and asked her why she didn't immediately get screened, she agreed she should have, knowing that the cancer would take her life. But then she said something that had never crossed my mind.

"I was afraid you might not be attracted to me anymore if I had to have a breast removed," she said. "I know how much you like my breasts and all."

Yikes! I could not believe what I just heard. Was this all my fault? Was I so addicted to her breasts that she would risk her life to keep me aroused?

She was quick to tell me that the fault was completely hers, and that she knew she should have gone immediately after finding that small lump. She said she knew I would have still loved her with or without her breasts. And while that is true, there were three profound questions that hit me right in the face with her words:

Was I too focused on sex and her breasts?
As much as I fondled her breasts, how was it that I didn't find that lump?
Why didn't I notice Becky was sick for that year before her diagnosis?

Even to this day, I live with the guilt that I should have known. As men, aren't we supposed to protect our wives? While the responsibility was Becky's to take care of her body, I can't help but believe I bear some of the blame. I should have known, but I didn't, which is why I have written this book. So that you will not make the same mistakes that I did.

The biggest failing for me though, was that I knew little about breast cancer. To me, breast cancer was just a pink ribbon on an NFL football in October. This disease only attacked other women, not my wife. Had I known then what I know now that — those breasts I loved so much were not just arousing orbs, but also ticking timebombs — Becky might still be alive today.

In the next chapter, we begin our journey to a full understanding of this terrible disease and how we, as guys, can actually play a positive role in preventing breast cancer in the women we love.

Chapter Two
A Practical Definition of "The Breast"

"Living is Easy with Eyes Closed."
— **John Lennon**

In order to be fully prepared for and aware of this disease, we need to have a deeper understanding of *the breast;* so let's take a biological look at this pleasurable part of our lover's anatomy to begin our journey in understanding this disease.

The breast is a tissue overlying the chest (pectoral) muscles. It is made of a specialized tissue that produces milk as well as fatty tissue. The amount of fat determines the size of the breast.

The milk-producing part of the breast is organized into 15 to 20 sections called *lobes*. Within each lobe are smaller structures, called *lobules,* where the milk is produced. The milk travels through a network of tiny tubes called *ducts*. The ducts connect and come together into larger ducts, which eventually exit the skin in the nipple. The dark area of skin surrounding the nipple is called the areola.

Connective tissue and ligaments provide support to the breast and give it its shape. Nerves provide sensation to the breast. The breast also contains blood vessels, lymph vessels, and lymph nodes.

Ok, now let's be honest. Did you know any of this? Oh sure, you knew about the nipple, and the nerves and the sensation your woman feels, but did you know that the breast was so complex? I am not afraid to admit that when Becky got sick, I didn't know most of this.

There are many different types of breasts too, information that we, as guys, don't really need to know about. But, what we do need is to know, and know well, is our wife's breasts. You can do the self-check for her. If something looks slightly different on one of her breasts, tell her. Don't wait! Bring this to her attention immediately.

On my wedding night with Becky, as I looked at her breasts, I noticed that the left one was just ever so slightly deformed. Nothing big, but different from her other one. I could tell that she was very self-conscience about it, so I never actually asked her about it, or what happened. Yet the exact place where her small lump the size of a BB first formed was in the area that was slightly deformed. Coincidence? I will never know, because I did not force her to see her oncologist. I didn't want to embarrass her.

In the next chapter, Dr. Carla Garcia, one of our country's foremost experts on breast cancer, will dig into the causes and types of breast cancer. But first, I want to go back and take a deeper dive into what we examined in Chapter One, especially now that we have a very different understanding of the breast.

As guys, we all know we are obsessed with, maybe even addicted to, women's breasts. One way we see this obsession is the huge vocabulary guys use when discussing them: boobs, jugs, hooters, melons, headlights, fun bags, globes, knobs, ta-tas, mammaries, chest toys, the girls, and on and on it goes. Personally, I was shocked when I researched the various names that guys have attributed to breasts, and I suppose I was a bit offended as well. Just seems like such disrespect to the woman. Maybe this is because when Becky got sick, her breasts took on a very different meaning to me; or could be that I'm just old school.

This disrespect for women's breasts is all throughout our culture. Just ask any waitress. She will tell you that low-cut tops that expose some cleavage means better tips. How many women have complained that in conversations with men, the guys look at their breasts, not their faces? Have you done this? I know I have. I have had women tell me that if they are applying for a job, they believe that being "highly qualified" is not as important as having the "biggest breasts" if their boss is a man. Kind of makes the man look shallow, doesn't it?

Just as some women look for a certain body type or height in men, some guys look for a certain breast size in women. But most men like *all* breasts, especially those that are attached to the women they're involved with.

UCLA and Cal State Los Angeles found in an online survey of 52,227 heterosexual adults, ages 18 to 65, that 56 percent said they were "satisfied with their partners' breasts," which means that 44 percent of men — a large proportion — feel *unsatisfied*. Many women who get augmented say their husband or boyfriend encouraged or pressured them into it. Shame on those guys.

In this same study among women, only 30 percent felt satisfied with their own breasts. The researchers observed: "Younger and thinner women worried that their breasts were too small. Older and heavier women were concerned about droopiness."

In fact, 70 percent of women — almost three-quarters — say they're dissatisfied with their breasts and many of them take action. Countless millions of women wear padded bras or choose fashions that will focus the man's attention away from or toward their breasts, depending on how they feel about their chests.

Breast surgery is the number one cosmetic procedure in the U.S. today. The American Society of Plastic Surgery estimates that every year American women undergo some 400,000 breast augmentations and 150,000 breast reductions. Women who get augmented typically want a cup or two increase, most typically from A or B to C. Women who want reductions typically go one or two cup sizes down.

Ok, I think I have made my point.

As I wrote in Chapter One, I still wonder if my obsession and addiction to Becky's breasts caused her to ignore that very small lump she found, afraid that I might not love her anymore if she had to have it removed to spare her life. She did ignore it and it did take her life.

I understand that as guys, our breast obsession is clearly sexual and that our woman's breasts are among our favorite sex toys. This is normal and healthy for intimacy.

I'm just saying that we all must be very careful going forward about how much attention and value we place on our woman's breasts. We don't want to be the reason she is dissatisfied with her chest, and we certainly don't want her to hide from us any irregularity that may occur in either breast — that could change your lives forever.

At the risk of losing our flow, I am going to switch gears a bit for the next two chapters because I think it is important for you to hear from two people who are very powerful experts in their fields.

Chapter Three is written by Dr. Carla Garcia, D.O.M., a well-recognized authority on breast screening and my foundation's Medical Director, in addition to just being a really cool and smart lady! She will tell us how breast cancer starts and where breast cancer comes from.

Chapter Four is written by Mr. Khevin Barnes whose expertise is that he survived breast cancer. Yep, guys get breast cancer too, which is the title of his chapter. His story is a powerful one!

I promise I will be back for Chapter Five through the end of the book because there is still so much we have to do.

Please know that by contributing a chapter to my book, neither Dr. Garcia nor Khevin necessarily endorse my opinions, viewpoints, or beliefs. We only need to agree on one thing: Preventing breast cancer, which we all do, wholeheartedly.

Chapter Three
How Does It Start and Where Does It Come From?

by Dr. Carla Garcia

"Without education, we are in a horrible and deadly danger of taking educated people seriously."
— **G.K. Chesterton**

Before writing this chapter, Rick was kind enough to send me his outline and the first chapters you have probably finished reading. This was particularly helpful since it is a "Guy's Guide," and women do not always understand men's thinking (and vice versa). Numerous books have been written about this discrepancy in how the sexes process information and communicate, but it has not improved our understanding of gender mentality by any measurable quantity. So let me say at this beginning of my writing: "The opinions expressed by the male authors of this book are not necessarily my own."

Rick's kind introduction is appreciated but I don't consider myself an expert on breast cancer. I am a doctor who has been doing breast exams and breast screenings for over 20 years, and I have seen thousands of women, and a couple of men, with breast cancer.

Rick has explained that Becky did not get a breast screening, even after finding a lump in her breast. Why not? Because there are five words we all repeat to ourselves when we are worried about an impending health problem — "maybe it will go away." So we wait to get it checked, and because we don't know how long we should wait, we wait too long. In fact, a few days after beginning to write this chapter, a family member was diagnosed with bilateral breast cancer. Yep, my family member was diagnosed with cancer in both breasts. She had not done a breast screening in 10 years, but her massage therapist found it during a massage appointment and encouraged her to get it checked.

How does breast cancer start? Well, if we knew the answer to that question, we could prevent it from ever developing. We don't catch cancer like we say we "catch a cold." It is not contagious. We don't inherit cancer — less than 10% of cancers have a genetic component. So, what happens when we develop cancer? There is no single answer. Some say it is sex hormones and some say it is environmental toxins. Physicians can't agree on whether obesity, eating a high fat diet, or drinking alcohol causes breast cancer. BUT…there is one thing that everyone agrees on and that is that exercise helps prevent cancer — all types of cancer.

At this point, I usually tell my patients to let "the girls" exercise. I say:
a. Don't wear a bra for more than 12 hours a day.
b. Reduce the use of underwire bras. When you wear an underwire bra the breasts can't bounce — they are in a cage. Remember that Rick said there is lymph in the breasts. The best way to move lymph is with exercise (bouncing). You can't take all underwire bras away from a stylish woman, but save them for dress-up and not for everyday wear.

c. Don't use anti-perspirants. Perspiration (sweat) clears out toxins. You can use a natural deodorant that does not contain aluminum or chemicals that prevent perspiration.

d. Finally, I recommend "rebounding." Rebounding for just 3 minutes a day moves the lymph more than any other form of exercise.

So, what happens to make a tumor form? Basically, our bodies are made up of cells. These cells die off and are replaced by new cells. If the number of new cells is more than the number of dying cells, a mass of cells called a tumor can form. In essence our bodies maintain a delicate balance between the old and the new. A **healthy** immune system should keep the destruction and creation of cells in balance.

Not all tumors are malignant (cancerous). In fact, the majority of breast lumps are not cancerous. More often than not they are fluid-filled cysts or lumps composed of fibroid tissue (these are called fibroadenomas). A friend of mine had a lump in her breast that would come and go. She associated it with the amount of coffee she was drinking so she named her lump "Jean" after a brand of coffee she was particularly fond of. I would hear her say "Well Jean is being a pain today," only to have people ask her who "Jean" was.

Does coffee cause breast cysts? Probably not, but many of us are deficient in the enzyme that metabolizes caffeine properly, so it can become an irritant to breast tissue. A lot of times cysts will diminish with decreased caffeine consumption. I never tell anybody to quit caffeine "cold turkey"; the withdrawals can cause headaches, mood swings, and general "witchyness." You know what I am talking about; many of us do not want to talk until we've had our morning coffee.

How can you tell the difference between a cyst and a concerning lump? Cysts are movable, soft, and somewhat round. Lumps that should be clinically evaluated are hard, immovable, and have irregular borders (sharp edges). You and your spouse/lover are encouraged to feel for lumps. The majority of women who come in for breast screening have either found a lump by doing a self-breast exam, or their partner has felt it and become concerned. Don't believe for a second that you "don't know what you are doing." Breast exams are not rocket science. The best thing is to perform regular breast exams (palpations) so that you know what the breast feels like normally. You will know if you feel the breasts regularly when something changes or feels different and that it is time to get a second opinion, preferably by a licensed medical professional.

There is no exact science to breast palpations. That is palpation NOT palpitation (irregular heartbeat). Try to do it once a month, at a time when she is not on her menstrual cycle. Hormone fluctuations that accompany the menstrual cycle can cause cysts and lumps to come and go.

Look at the breasts. Look for changes in size, shape, puckering, dimpling, or discoloration.

1. Feel for changes in the breast. Use the pads of your fingers and do not apply too much pressure. (Too little pressure and you won't be doing a good breast exam.) Your fingers should stay in constant contact with the breast, so that you don't miss a "spot." In other words, do not lift your fingers off the breast to move to a

different area. You can look at the breast and imagine the face of a clock where you start at 12:00 and go all around the "clock" in circles. That is the most commonly taught method. I find it easier to start at the collarbone and follow a straight line down to the infra-mammary (bra line directly under the breast) region. I feel the sternum (top to bottom), move my fingers over and feel top to bottom, repeating this until I have felt the entire breast. Don't forget to feel the underarms — there is a lot of lymph in those armpits.

2. Check the nipple for discharge. Clear or milky is common, greenish or pinkish should be checked. Any recent change in nipple discharge should be evaluated.

3. If you find a lump — don't panic! Get it checked. Do a breast screening with ultrasound, thermography, or mammography. Ask a health practitioner to do a palpation.

If you are ever faced with a breast cancer diagnosis it is not only frightening; it is confusing.

There are stages and grades and types (Oh my)! Rick describes breast cancer stages in a later chapter, so I will try to summarize the different types of breast cancer.

DCIS (ductal carcinoma in situ) – This is thought of as a breast cancer in the very early stages and some have claimed it isn't cancer at all. Regardless of what anybody tells you about DCIS, treat it as though it is an early-stage cancer. DCIS is contained within the mild ducts (in situ). Survival rates are high, but it can lead to more invasive or aggressive cancers.

IDC (invasive ductal carcinoma) – It starts in the milk ducts but spreads to the surrounding breast tissue AND there are a bunch of different types of IDC.

There are so many types of breast cancer it can make your head spin: ILC, LCIS, molecular subtypes of breast cancer, phyllodes, and Paget's disease.

Here is the thing…not all breast cancers are lumps or tumors in the breast. Paget's disease starts on the nipple and can change the color of the areola. Inflammatory breast cancer is one of the most insidious types. It is an inflammation of the lining of the milk ducts. It is NOT usually seen on a mammogram or an ultrasound. Thermography, a camera that measures heat is one of the best ways to check for inflammatory breast disease.

Well, let's hope you never have to understand the types of breast cancer, because in addition to types there are hormonal and genetic classifications: HER2, estrogen positive, triple negative, and sundry other classes of breast cancer.

How can you prevent breast cancer? Well….you can eat a healthy diet, exercise, avoid stress (easier said than done), and do regular breast screenings. Studies have shown that supplementing with vitamin D3 can reduce the risk of breast cancer. Limit the exposure to ionizing radiation, such as x-rays. Yes, mammograms are x-rays and sometimes they are necessary but try to space them out and do ultrasound or thermography in between to limit radiation exposure. It gets complicated because insurance does not cover thermography and it doesn't usually pay for an ultrasound unless you do a mammogram.

Lastly let me say that the most important thing you can do is support your loved one's decisions with regards to her treatment. Friends and family will come out of the woodwork with treatments, supplements, and "expert" opinions. They have the best of intentions but once you hear the word "cancer" in your diagnosis it is overwhelming and "chatter" from those around you is NOT helpful.

Recovering from cancer is a very personal journey. Nobody can walk in the cancer patient's shoes, but they can walk beside them with love and encouragement. I have seen patients live beyond a "terminal" diagnosis, myself included. These "survivors" had faith, took control of their health by changing their diet and exercise routines, adopted a positive attitude, and embraced social support (this is where you come in — be their support). Although it is her diagnosis, it will affect you and those closest to you. On the other side of the spectrum, I have seen patients die from untreated DCIS (you know…the early-stage cancer mentioned above). These patients were fatalistic, let others decide what their treatments should be, and did not have a strong will to go on living and most importantly they did not have emotional or social support.

Some of my patients have used natural modalities, some have done surgery, some have done chemotherapy or radiation, and some have done a combination of both natural and conventional medicine. It is not my job to judge their choices — nor is it yours. This is about the person with the diagnosis. We can help them evaluate their options, but the ultimate decision for treatments are with the patient being treated. When we are faced with our own diagnosis (and let's pray that never happens), we can choose for ourselves what the best treatment is for us. Hopefully, there is somebody like you (the reader) that will walk alongside us, with love and encouragement and patience.

Dr. Carla Garcia is a board-certified Doctor of Oriental Medicine in New Mexico with more than 20 years of experience in Thermography. She has performed thousands of scans in the U.S. and Canada. She has trained in the United States and Germany and is certified as a Clinical Thermographer by the American College of Clinical Thermology, the only Non-Profit, Medical Thermography Board in the United States. Contact Dr. Carla at ThermographyNM@aol.com.

Chapter Four
Men Get Breast Cancer Too?

by Khevin Barnes, Survivor

The courage we desire and prize is not the courage to die decently, but to live manfully.
—**Thomas Carlyle**

On May 11, 2014, I received a message on my cell phone from the surgeon who had, just days before, performed a needle biopsy on a tiny lump in my left breast. I had flown from Hawaii to California to say goodbye to my ninety-three-year-old mother who, with compromised health, had broken her hip and was not expected to live more than a few days. Ironically for both of us, it was "Mother's Day."

"Hi Khevin. I have a bit of bad news. The breast mass is cancer..."

The message on my phone was brief and to the point, and I can still replay it my mind years later. There were a few quiet words, an apology with a hint of disappointment, and suddenly my life was changed forever.

I was a man with breast cancer.

Most men I talk with are surprised when they hear that guys can actually contract cancer in their breasts. It's an "orphan disease," meaning that it's understudied, largely overlooked, and unabashedly ignored by the pharmaceutical industry because there's no money to be made here.

Frustrating as that may be, I understand that's how the world works. In the words of Mr. Spock of Star Trek fame, as he took a huge dose of deadly radiation in order to save the crew of his star ship, *"The needs of the many outweigh the needs of the few—or the one."* And so, we are a small but increasingly vocal group of cancer survivors, intent on letting the world know that male breast cancer is real.

When I was diagnosed at the age of 64, the odds of a male contracting breast cancer were 1000 to 1. Statistically, a man was more likely to accidentally drown in any given year than he was to contract cancer in his breast. That wasn't exactly reassuring news, but at least it put my disease in perspective. Guys represent just 1% of all breast cancer cases.

Male breast cancer found me while I was a full-time resident at the Palolo Zen Center in Honolulu, Hawaii. My wife and I had been practicing Zen Meditation for many years, and after retiring from my work on stage as a professional magician, the thought of continuing our practice in Hawaii for twelve months while living in a Zen Buddhist Temple was a dream come true for both of us.

As you can imagine, life was simple there. We ate vegetarian meals, studied the teachings of Zen, sat every day in meditation, worked in the gardens, and walked on the beach. But still I got cancer.

I suppose that's proof that a healthy lifestyle in paradise is no guarantee of a healthy life.

But if Zen taught me anything, it's that stuff happens, and we can choose how we react to challenging moments in our lives. Naturally I was alarmed, frightened, and surprised by this cancer I never knew existed; but I was also very aware that I was alive at that moment and needed to carefully consider my game plan while preparing for the possibility that my time on Earth could be seriously shortened.

After my mastectomy surgery, I was diagnosed with stage one, grade three breast cancer. Grade three indicates a fast growing and aggressive form of the disease, but stage one means that the tumor is contained, and that's a good thing. Most males are found to have a more advanced degree of the disease, and that's only because we are slow when it comes to getting help with what many men still think of as "a woman's disease." In general, guys find it more difficult to speak up when we find a body part out of whack. Diagnosis and treatment procedures are disconcerting for many men as well, and men are more likely to attribute a symptom such as a breast lump to some other cause.

I was fortunate to catch my cancer early. But I had some help. A few days before my diagnosis I was visiting my primary care physician in Honolulu for a routine visit, and as I was getting up to leave he asked, "Is there anything else going on that we should talk about?"

"No!" I replied, puffing up my proverbial, masculine chest to which my wife, who was at my side, chimed in, "Honey, why don't you show him that little bump in your breast?" Painless and about the size of a pea, I had discovered it while taking a shower a few weeks earlier. I was scheduled for a mammogram the next day, followed by an ultra sound and needle biopsy a few days later, and I was in surgery for a mastectomy of my left breast less than thirty days after that conversation.

The swiftness of those events by my sharp-eyed doctor and determined wife probably saved my life.

Information on cancer of the male breast is scarce, and few doctors routinely check for it. And when it is diagnosed, the standard course of treatment recommended is often the same as that for women, since there isn't a lot of historical data to guide us. There are a number of healthcare professionals who question the effectiveness of many of these treatments, and new research has shown that men do indeed react differently to traditional chemotherapies such as Tamoxifen.

Even with all the medical help from surgeons and oncologists, not to mention the unending advice we are certain to get from our concerned friends and family members, the choices we make are ultimately our own, and they are never easy. After all, a cancer diagnosis is an expedition in extremes. It shatters every thought and plan we have about our future, and leaves us with many more questions than answers. It is at once a mind-gripping nightmare into a world of the unknown and an auspicious gift, provoking us to gather our lives, confront our vulnerabilities, and discover our strengths.

I sought out the opinions of several oncologists to aid me in plotting my plan of action. But with a rare cancer that offered little in the way of research, clinical trials, or pharmaceutical support, I found myself making some tough decisions on my own. Statistically, with my form of breast cancer, I was given an 80% chance of surviving for five years, and in the end, those odds were good enough for me. Other than my annual mammogram, I chose to decline any further medical intervention.

Cancer requires that we make a series of highly personal and consequential choices, and once I had made mine, I was ready to move ahead with my life. And I was determined to take an active role in my own health and healing while helping the other men who were certain to follow in my footsteps. I began writing for several cancer magazines, wrote and composed a stage musical about male breast cancer, and spoke to audiences of both women and men who had breast cancer too. Not surprisingly, there were not too many men in attendance.

The similarities and differences in breast cancer for women and men are subtle, but measurable. After all, we may be divided in our anatomy, but at the end of the day, and despite the sea of pink that surrounds us, breast cancer really is a genderless disease. It's my hope that we can find a way to become color coordinated and work together to eliminate all breast cancers from our lives.

For men experiencing breast cancer, it's sometimes a struggle to feel included in the march toward an eventual cure. After all, the stigmas about breasts are centuries long. Understandably, the thought of a woman losing one or both breasts to cancer is disconcerting to say the least. Female breasts have long been symbolic of fertility and well-being. There isn't much in the way of symbolism or adulation to attach to the male version.

I think the greatest hope for men to come out of the shadow of breast cancer in a very pink world is through the support from women. The avenues of education are already in place. The clinical trials, long favoring the female participants, are slowly being cracked open to include men. Male breast cancer survivors don't need a pink pass to join in with this crusade of life and longevity which, after all, is the ultimate goal of every cancer survivor around the world.

SO WHAT CAN MEN DO?

Guys have to take matters into their own hands. Literally. We need to get used to feeling our chests and under our arms regularly, keeping an eye out for any unusual changes, no matter how innocuous they may seem. Thirty seconds in the shower should do the trick. And we ought to get comfortable with the fact that we are aging. And as we age, we open ourselves to changes in our bodies, not all of them good. Early detection is always a good thing however. Breast cancer is no more a woman thing than being an astronaut, a firefighter, or the leader of a country is a man thing. The times have changed and so too has medicine and science and human awareness.

But make no mistake. Guys are still a small piece of the proverbial pie when it comes to breast cancer awareness. There is a pink connection that influences everything we do, and naturally it's the overwhelming numbers of women diagnosed with the disease who create this disparity between male and female breast cancers. It's no fault of theirs, of course. I wholeheartedly support the women with breast cancer. But it will require the incessant ambition from guys to add their voices to the mix. It will take **T**ime, **I**nformation, **D**edication, and **E**ducation to influence what I like to call the changing "**T.I.D.E**." of male breast cancer.

Male breast cancer is a disease that can leave us feeling alone and vulnerable with its perilous challenges. But we're all mountain climbers in a sense, and men and women are on the very same expedition to wellness. If we choose to climb up and into the experience of survival, meeting the challenges with patience, determination, and a bit of courage, it can offer us a wider view of our own place in the world. And as we push onward and upward step by step, we may realize that this journey could take our lives at any moment or, with a bit of luck, infuse us with the greatest inspiration to live in new and remarkable ways.

Khevin Barnes is a male breast cancer survivor, playwright, stage magician, and musician. He is the writer/composer of a new musical about Male Breast Cancer called "THE SONS OF SAINT AGATHA" and is currently searching for a producer or two to sponsor the show in a national tour.

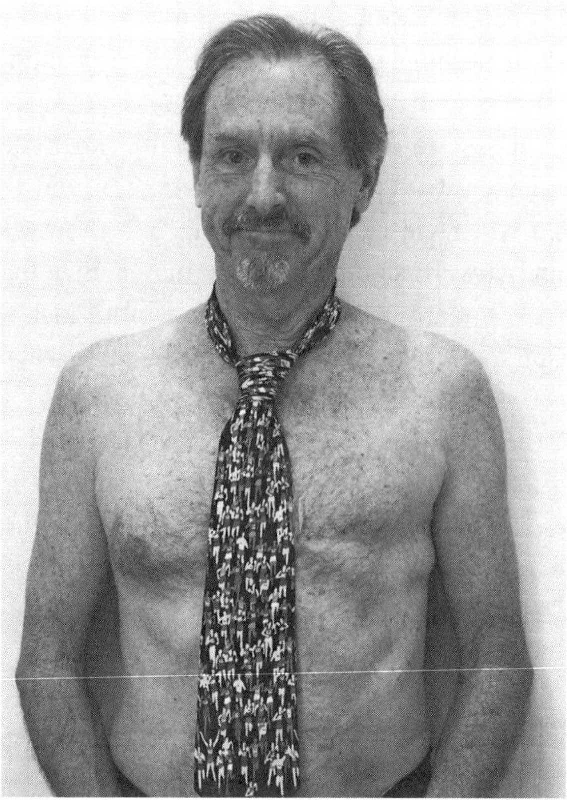

Chapter Five
The Man and The Mammogram

It is easier to find men who will volunteer to die, than to find those who are willing to endure pain with patience.
—**Julius Caesar**

A special thanks to Dr. Carla Garcia and Khevin Barnes for their invaluable contribution to this book. I am sure you were fascinated by Khevin's story, as was I.

As I read about his incredible journey, and how today he has become such a strong advocate for male breast cancer detection and prevention, I was reminded of a conversation I had recently with my UBER driver.

His name is Bob Noble and he asked me about the Becky Baker Foundation logo on the golf cap I was wearing. I told him that my foundation provides free mammograms and thermograms for those who cannot afford the screening, and he asked me how many mammograms I had given away to men. I told him of the 2,400 or so we have provided in the past three years, only about 100 were for men. He then said, "I had a mammogram and wrote a short story about my horrific experience. Would you like to read it?"

I couldn't wait!

He emailed it to me and gave me permission to publish, so I wanted to include it here for my "guy" readers. I hope you like it as much as I do.

I am a 49-year-old white male, 245 lbs, 6'1" and uh, not physically active. There, I said it. I have a sedentary job, driving charter buses out of Palm Springs, CA. Since retiring from the military nine years ago, I've sort of let my body go. This past May, I was surprised to find a large lump under my left armpit.

At first, I passed it off as just a fatty deposit, nothing more. Eventually, though, it started to hurt. Not all the time, but when the pain came, I took notice. When I asked my loving wife to look at the lump, she actually gasped! (Oops, maybe this is more serious than I thought.) At her insistence, I made an appointment with our family physician.

The P.A. (physician's assistant) is the one who took my case; a perky, petite, no-nonsense female. She examined the lump, asked several questions, then mentioned that my left breast looked about 30% larger to her than my right breast. (Uh, have I gotten large enough to have breasts?!) With her medical experience, she suggested I get a couple different procedures done, just in case. To ease my fears, she mentioned it could be anything from an inflamed sweat gland to an enlarged lymph node to male breast cancer. The two tests (a mammogram and an ultrasound) would help rule out male breast cancer.

I have just returned from the torture that is passed off as a mammogram.

Ladies, I tip my hat to you. I'm not sure how you can do this procedure on a yearly basis, knowing full well the incredible pain that awaits you. I have just endured my first (and, I pray, ONLY) *mammogram. Having completed this procedure, I can say with only a slight exaggeration that I would enjoy a vasectomy, without anesthesia, rather than endure another mammogram. It begs the question: who tolerates a mammogram better? The buxom female or the slightly-built lady? I have never felt such pain as having my breast tissue squashed between 2 plates of glass, for the purpose of taking pictures. At no time did they mention whether they wanted wallet-sized or 8x10 glossies! Just when you think the attendant has mashed your breast tissue as flat as humanly possible, they ratchet the vice about three notches tighter, then have the nerve to tell you to not move or breathe.*

Male breast cancer is a very real, though rare, disease. I'm happy that my P.A. was willing to take precautions for my health. I only trust that it is something far less severe than male breast cancer. I hope to never experience a mammogram again as long as I live. Now, if you will excuse me, I'm going to put 2 ice packs on my chest…

Good news, Bob's lump was not breast cancer, and while he might have exaggerated his pain associated with the procedure, he did what was necessary to take care of his body.

Don't want to endure a mammogram or the compression? Schedule a thermogram. No pain, just a high-resolution picture from a camera similar to what's attached to our satellites that can be as far as 23,000 miles out in space and still read the logo on your shirt.

Regardless, if you feel a lump of any size, schedule your screening today!

Chapter Six
Will There Ever Be a Cure?

"Once you choose hope, anything's possible."
— **Christopher Reeve**

We've all seen advertisements and articles claiming that there is a "cure" for breast cancer. They flood the Internet, some authored by major publications, and others written by quacks who believe if you eat a certain type of tree bark, you will be cured of breast cancer. Trust me, Becky ate this bark, and it did not cure her breast cancer.

The well-known website *wikiHow.com* has even jumped into the cure game with an article published just last year entitled, "How to Cure Breast Cancer." Yep, that's the actual title and so this is one of the first articles that appears when you do an Internet search for "curing breast cancer."

It details seven "methods" for curing breast cancer, with not a one an actual cure. The title is misleading, and the article has little to do with "curing" breast cancer, spending most of its words talking about medical treatment, surgery, chemo, and scheduling regular screening visits. The authors are very loose with their definition of the word "cure," implying that if the chemo kills the breast cancer, you have been cured.

There are literally hundreds of these articles online, many of them as misleading as the *wikiHow* article.

On the other end of the curing spectrum, we have the natural cure websites. One of these is earthclinic.com and they have published articles claiming that supplements such as Turmeric, Flaxseed, Calcium, and even Baking Soda, may actually cure breast cancer. These are all great supplements (not sure about baking soda) and might indeed help to *prevent* breast cancer, but there is no evidence that these or the many other supplements that are out there will "cure" breast cancer.

Probably the most well-known event that is associated with curing breast cancer in the U.S. is the "Run For The Cure."

These 5K runs are held all throughout the U.S. and attract tens of thousands of runners each year. Most of these participants have somehow been affected by this evil disease and want to show their support for finding the cure to breast cancer. They may be survivors or have had a loved one or friend lose their fight with the disease.

Many breast cancer foundations sponsor a "Run For The Cure," and for those guys who don't really pay too much attention to these races, they may think that, one, these races are bringing about a cure for breast cancer, and two, all the money raised at these charity events goes to diligently searching for a "cure."

They would be wrong on both counts. In fact, little of the money raised at these events ever actually goes toward finding a cure.

Here is a statement from the website of Susan G. Komen, one of the largest breast cancer foundations and the one that actually started these races. Read it closely and see if you can spot the word that is missing:

"The Susan G. Komen Race for the Cure is an education and fundraising event for breast cancer. The series of 5K runs and fitness walks raises significant funds and awareness for the breast cancer movement, celebrates breast cancer survivorship and honors those who have lost their battle with the disease."

Now, did you catch what is missing from their official statement? Yep, it's the word "cure."

The logical question then is, where does all this money go if not to "finding a cure?" When you have an hour, spend some time on the Komen website and see if you can follow where the money goes. But, be prepared to be disappointed.

The Canadian Cancer Society also has their curing event that they call "Never Stop Running for The Cure."

In Canada, breast cancer is the leading cause of cancer deaths and they have mobilized a massive group of supporters who give and participate annually to help find a cure.

In 2019, they had over 85,000 participants and raised $17 million in communities across Canada. Here is their official statement about this event from their website:

This event unites an incredible collective of Canadians who are a force-for-life in the face of breast cancer and want to show their support. It's an inspirational day that raises significant funds for CCS, the largest charitable funder of breast cancer research in Canada. CCS invests these dollars into ground-breaking breast cancer research, compassionate support services, trusted cancer information and advocacy on behalf of all Canadians. It's because of the funds Canadians raise through the CIBC Run for the Cure that we know more than ever before about how to prevent, diagnose, treat and live with and beyond breast cancer.

Notice what word is missing from their last sentence? Yep, it's that same testy word "cure." If this *Run* was truly about "curing breast cancer" their final sentence would read:

It's because of the funds Canadians raise through the CIBC Run for the Cure that we know more than ever before about how to cure, prevent, diagnose, treat and live with and beyond breast cancer.

The CCS did not hold their run in 2020 due to COVID, instead opting for this message on their website:

Our reimagined CIBC Run for the Cure may be over, but it's not too late to help change the future of breast cancer. Our website will be accepting online donations until December 31. Together, we can continue to show Canadians facing breast cancer that we will never stop running.

"Donations" for what, exactly?
Unfortunately, many breast cancer foundations in the U.S. are not much different.

Look, it's not my purpose to condemn these foundations, many of which are ethical and transparent with their mission. I only want you to

Charlie at 4 weeks.

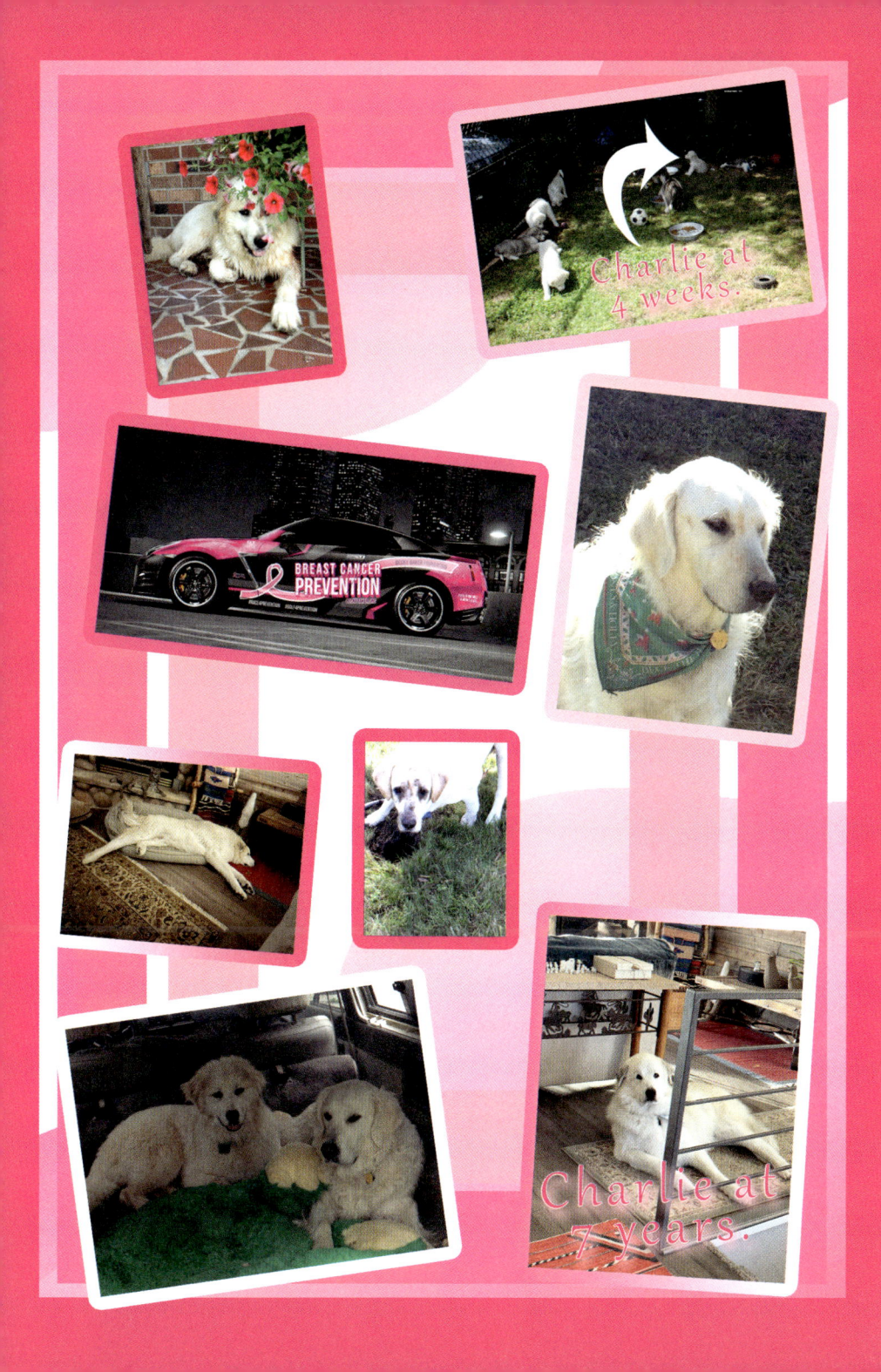

Charlie at 7 years.

Miss Penny, at 3 Months

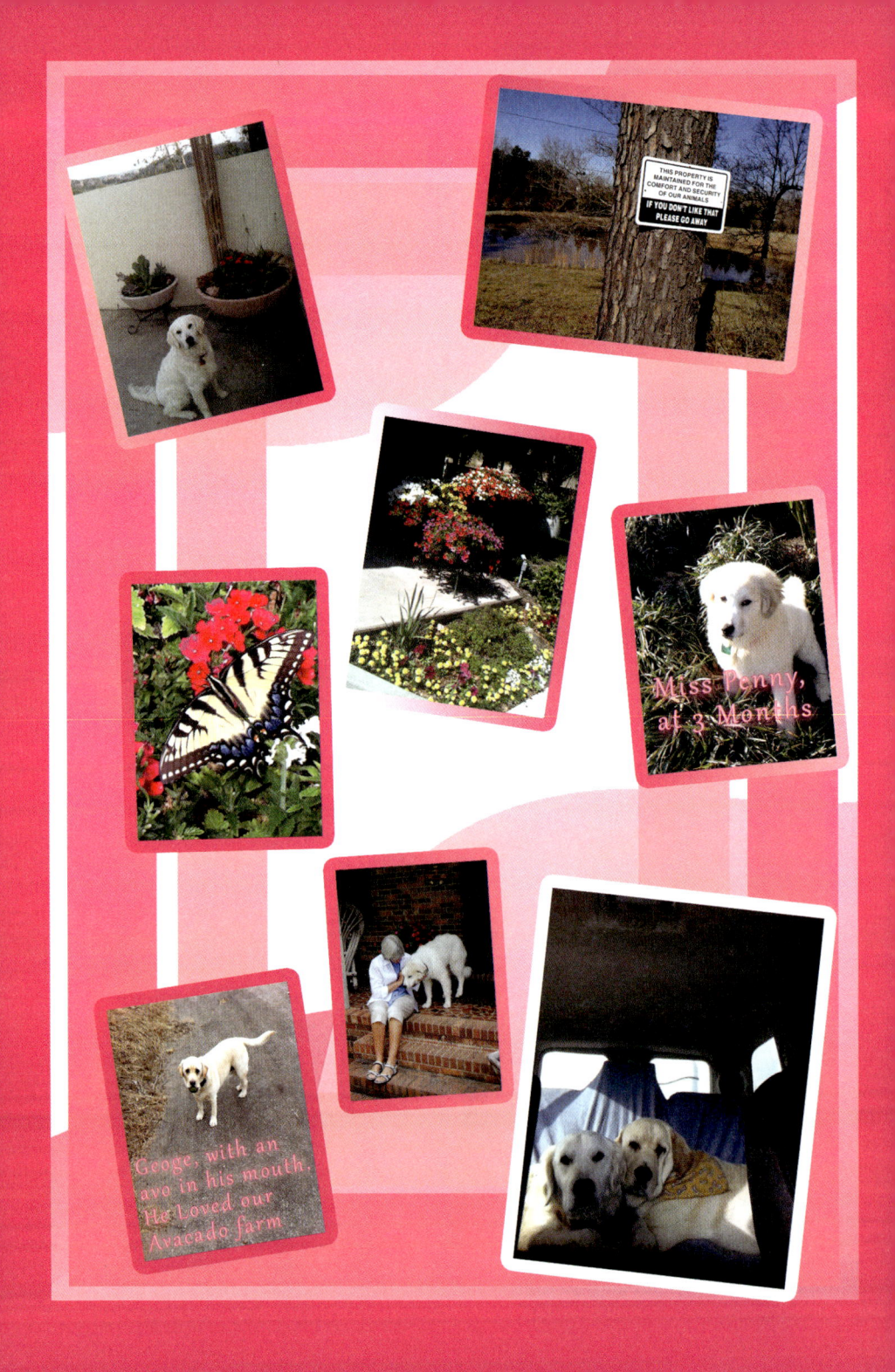

Geoge, with an avo in his mouth, He Loved our Avacado farm

With Hoover on Hilton Head Island

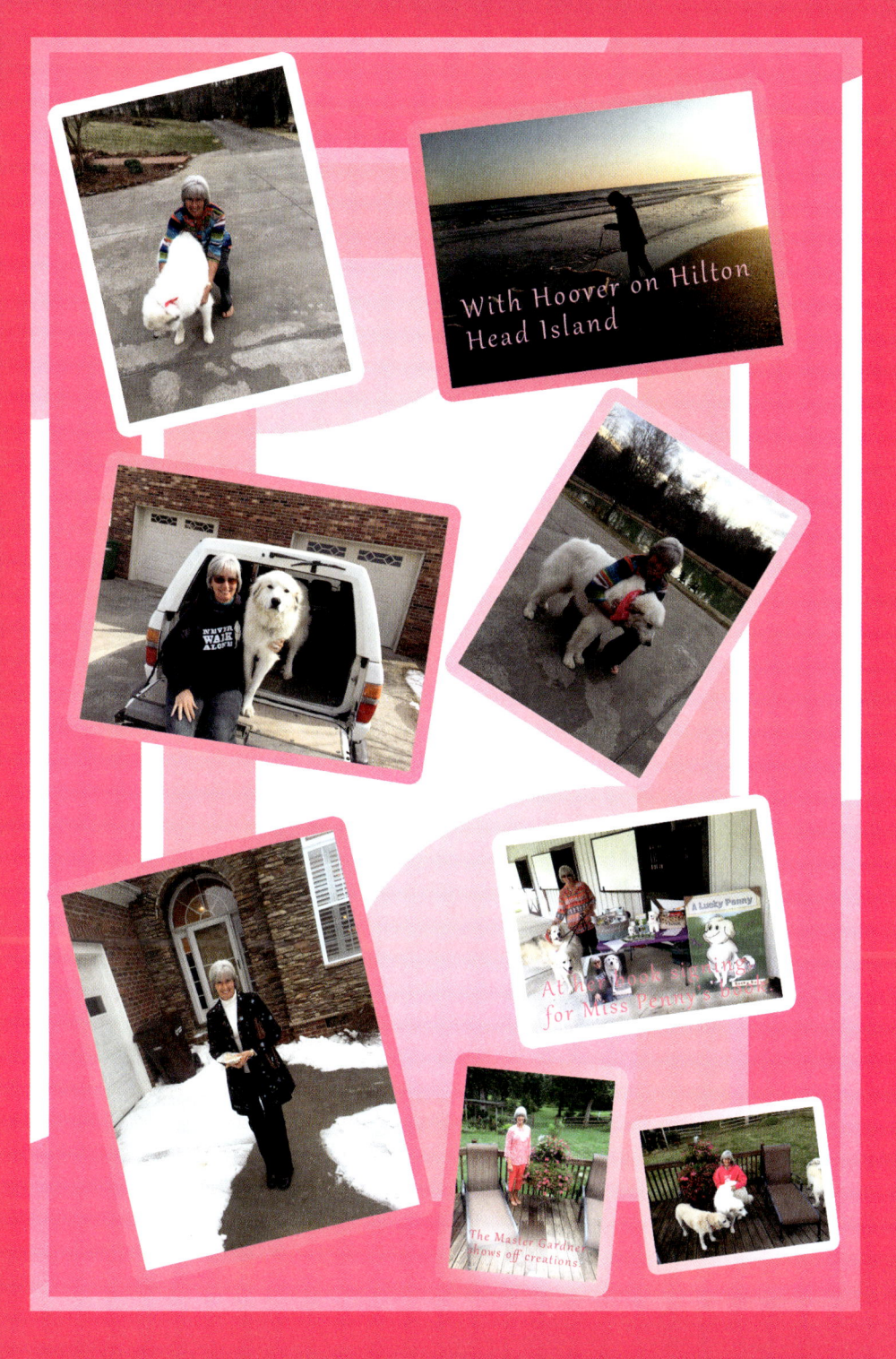

At the Look-Up for Miss Penny's

The Master Gardner shows off creations

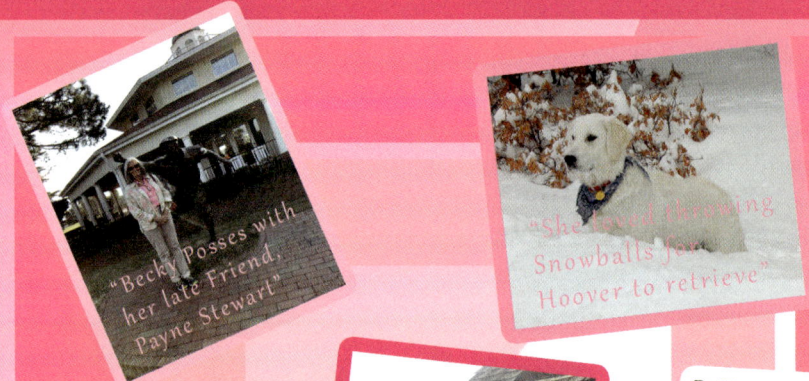

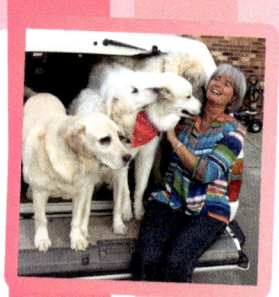

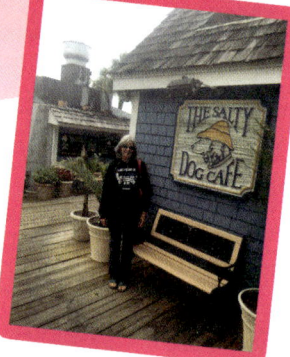

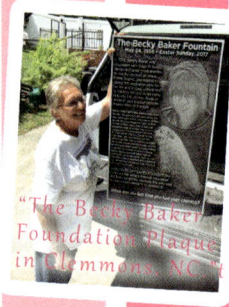

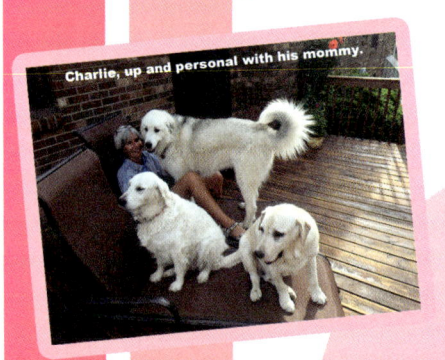

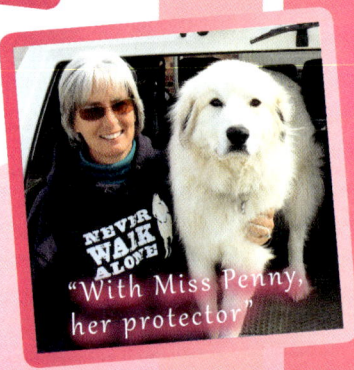

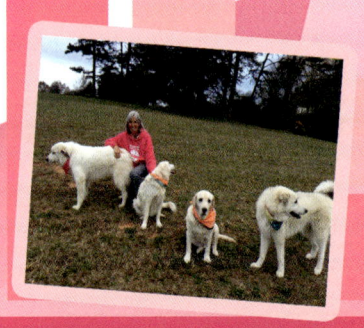

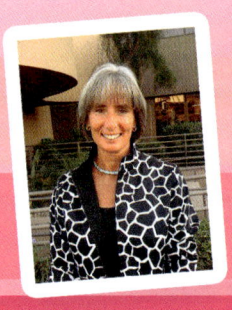

"Becky Posses with her late Friend, Payne Stewart"

"She loved throwing Snowballs for Hoover to retrieve"

"The Becky Baker Foundation Plaque in Clemmons, NC"

Charlie, up and personal with his mommy.

"With Miss Penny, her protector"

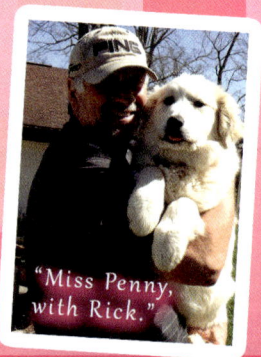

"Miss Penny, with Rick."

be aware that the breast cancer industry raises many billions of dollars annually on their claim that a "cure for breast cancer is right around the corner," and there is nothing wrong with you or I questioning their motives, especially when they ask for our support.

Simply put, if these organizations sponsor a Run For The Cure, then these funds need to go toward finding a cure, period.

But what about a cure for breast cancer? Will there ever be one anytime soon?

Nope. That's according to the honest scientists, who say that we should not count on a cure in the near or far future. Instead, they say we should find a way to live with it.

Dr. Jørgen Olsen is head of research at The Danish Cancer Society, and he says that any claim that a cure for breast cancer is "right round the corner" is a "far cry from reality."

"I think it's an illusion to imagine that after millions of years of this disease we'll suddenly find a solution. I don't think that we'll ever beat it, but I think that we'll get it under control so that it becomes chronic but not deadly," says Olsen.

Prominent cancer researcher, Mads Daugaard from the Molecular Pathology & Cell Imaging Laboratory at the University of British Colombia, Canada, agrees.

"We won't find a cure, but we'll probably reach a point where we have so many ways to attack cancer that people won't die from it anymore," says Daugaard.

Olsen suggests that "breast cancer could go from a deadly disease to a survivable one in around 10 to 14 years' time." Other types of cancer, such as cervical cancer, bowel cancer, lung cancer, throat cancer, and ovarian cancer might take a bit longer.

Many breast cancer foundations that seek to siphon off your hard-earned dollars won't tell you this fact. They are too busy trying to line their pockets with your donations to tell you the truth.

We aren't going to find a cure for breast cancer anytime soon, so maybe we stop donating to organizations who tell us they are "this close to finding the cure for breast cancer."

Instead of a Run for The Cure, how about a Run for Prevention? On average, only five to six percent of the annual 300,000+ breast cancer diagnoses in the U.S. are hereditary. This means, in theory anyway, that 94 to 95% of all cases are preventable.

Don't let anyone tell you that breast cancer is "not preventable."

The other day I was at my mailbox cluster when one of my neighbors, who is an MD, drove up to get his mail. We don't really know each other as our homes have some land between us and are not that close together. I was in the wrapped GTR and so he asked who Becky Baker was. I told him a bit about my foundation and my passion for preventing breast cancer.

He responded, "You can't prevent breast cancer." I have heard this statement many times before, usually from doctors. So, I used my standard example and talked about the man with lung cancer. I told him this man has stage IV and is near death. He started smoking at 20 years old, three packs a day for almost 50 years. The doctors tell him his lungs are burned so badly from his 50 years of smoking that he only has a short time left. I then asked my neighbor this question: 'If this man had not started smoking when he was 20 and had not smoked three packs a day for 50 years, do you think he would have lung cancer today?'

He said, "No." Like many doctors, he is a fatalist, and he is also very wrong. Breast cancer can be prevented.

We can prevent this evil disease. I always say that the best way to beat breast cancer is to not get it.

Chapter Seven
What About This Pink Ribbon?

"I like pink. It's just red's sorry, weak cousin."
— **Beth Fantaskey**

The Pink Ribbon.

We have all seen it, especially in October of each year when the nation transforms into "Breast Cancer Awareness Month."

In the NFL in October, the pink ribbons are everywhere. On footballs, the players' shoes, jerseys, and other memorabilia.

We see the pink ribbon plastered on merchandise at our local supercenter, usually with the words, "We support breast cancer," or, "A portion of the sale from this item goes to support breast cancer."

The pink ribbon is the official symbol of women's breast cancer and instantly identifies a breast cancer foundation that includes it in their logo. Seeing a pink ribbon, to some, validates the foundation as legit. To others, such as myself, the pink ribbon invites skepticism. We will talk more about this in the next chapter.

While the pink ribbon itself is not owned or trademarked by any single organization, many believe that the Susan G. Komen Foundation invented the pink ribbon, as it is usually first associated with their organization. Not true.

So, then, where did it come from?

Enter Charlotte Haley. In 1992 when she was battling breast cancer, she introduced the concept of a peach-colored breast cancer awareness ribbon.

The 68-year-old Haley began making peach ribbons by hand in her home. Many of her family members had breast cancer, including her grandmother, sister, and daughter.

So, to honor these family members, she began to distribute thousands of ribbons at local businesses with cards that read: "The National Cancer Institute's annual budget is $1.8 billion, only 5 percent goes for cancer prevention. Help us wake up our legislators and America by wearing this ribbon."

My kind of lady.

In no time at all, executives from Estée Lauder and Self Magazine asked Haley for permission to use her ribbon. We don't really know what their intentions were; all we know is that she refused. Which makes sense, knowing that her passion was exposing big corporations that cared more about the money than life. She didn't want her ribbon to be commercialized.

But Self Magazine would not take no for an answer, and as is the case with so many big corporations, wanted her ribbon whether she agreed or not. The magazine consulted its attorneys who told the executives the ribbon was Haley's, but suggested they change the color.

After consulting with many women around the country through surveys, they chose the color pink, because it is commonly viewed as "healing and soothing."

But, this disease is anything but soothing or healing.

Before Becky got sick, she was close to six feet tall and weighed 130 pounds. When she passed away, she was 5'8 and 60 pounds. Nothing "soothing" or "healing" about that. The metastatic ribbon color is black, which more accurately describes breast cancer and its effects on the body it consumes.

Soon, Charlotte Haley's peach ribbon was replaced with the pink ribbon, the same one we see today.

Many see the pink ribbon and immediately think of survivors, supporters, and organizations that are actively trying to end this disease.

I see the pink ribbon and think of fraud, which I address more in depth in the next chapter.

While my foundation does include a pink ribbon in its logo and marketing materials, I have made sure that my ribbon is a different shape and a deeper Pantone pink than the common ribbon everyone has seen.

I do this to try and distance myself as far as possible from these other foundations who spend the majority of their donations on their CEOs and other staff, rather than the person they claim to care about. I believe there is a special place in hell for anyone who raises money under the guise of curing breast cancer, all the while spending it on themselves or programs that have nothing to do with this disease. Komen is a perfect example — they were exposed for donating many thousands of dollars to Planned Parenthood for abortions, using funds that had been donated to them by unaware financial supporters. Many believe that Komen has still never recovered from this massive breach of trust.

Now you know why I dislike that pink ribbon so much, and why I have re-designed my ribbon. I refuse to be associated with other breast cancer foundations and have done everything possible to distance The Becky Baker Foundation from this money-grubbing industry.

We have been awarded the GuideStar Platinum Seal of Transparency every year we have been a 501(C)(3), which even Susan G. Komen cannot claim. My salary is $1 per year and close to ninety per cent of every dollar given goes toward providing a free screening to those who cannot afford the process. Still, it is a battle because everyday someone always seems to throw us in with these other conscienceless breast cancer foundations.

Chapter Eight
The Prostitution of The Pink Ribbon

*"If all you are doing is making money,
you have a luxurious but empty life."*
— **Amanda Donohoe**

By about September of each year, I start to become very unsettled. Why? Simple. Breast Cancer Awareness Month is just around the corner.

As I detailed in the last chapter, corporate America can't wait for this month every year. They see nothing but dollar signs, all earned on the back of this terrible disease.

In this chapter, I intend to expose Breast Cancer Awareness Month for what it really is: A racket. A rip-off. A shakedown. A sham.

It is my hope that you will then have a new understanding of the unintended consequences that are associated with this terrible annual campaign and not participate in it.

First, though, let's look at the history behind Breast Cancer Awareness Month.

In 1985, the American Cancer Society and the pharmaceutical division of Imperial Chemical Industries (now part of AstraZeneca, a leading manufacturer of oncology drugs) designated October as

National Breast Cancer Awareness Month. It was to be an observed commemorative month to raise awareness of breast cancer.

Claiming to "fill the information void" about breast cancer, the early mission of National Breast Cancer Awareness Month (NBCAM) was to educate and empower women to "take charge of their breast health."

The NBCAM website tells us that this designated October consists of "the creation and distribution of promotional materials, brochures, advertisements, public service spots, and other educational aids."

In addition to advertising, there is free exposure through word of mouth, clinical promotion, workplace and community initiatives, and political representatives. For years, the program encouraged routine self-breast exams and annual mammograms.

So, on the surface anyway, it looks as if the beginnings of this annual campaign were sincere. However, today's campaign is anything but. Let's examine it, in all its sordid details.

It starts the first day of October each year, when we will start to see online and at brick-and-mortar stores, all types of products marketed. From clothing to food to perfumes that have all been repackaged with a pink ribbon front and center.

They will imply, and often times boldly claim, that proceeds from the sale of these products will go to "Breast Cancer Awareness." These claims are outright lies.

This hustle is commonly called "Pinkwashing" and it's defined as:

Supporting the breast cancer cause or promoting a pink ribbon product while producing, manufacturing, and/or selling products linked to the disease. In recent years the definition has expanded to include any company or organization that exploits breast cancer for profit or public relations motivations.

Over the years "Pinkwasher" has become a common term used to describe the hypocrisy and lack of transparency that surrounds Breast Cancer Awareness Month and fundraising. It was coined by the group Breast Cancer Action in response to growing concerns about pink ribbon commercialization and the glut of pink ribbon products on the market.

Breast Cancer Action started calling out pinkwashers in 2002 as part of its *Think Before You Pink®* project, but their complaints have been largely drowned out by the sheer size of these corporations and their addiction to profit at any cost.

Today, with the ubiquity of cause-marketing and breast cancer promotions, many of us use the term pinkwasher to describe anyone who supports the breast cancer cause while profiting from the disease, or using it simply to enhance public relations.

Breast Cancer Action has called out everything from perfumes and body care products with known carcinogens or reproductive toxins to the use and manufacture of recombinant bovine growth hormone (rBGH) found in many dairy products and linked to cancer. Remember those famous Pink Buckets (of chicken) for the Cure? Yep, they had rBGH. I know, hard to believe.

Each year, corporations sell thousands of pink ribbon products with their own brand of awareness messages and fundraising promises. Yet many of these products contain chemicals linked to an increased risk of breast cancer, infertility, birth defects, and other health problems.

Why are these chemicals even on the market and do these corporations not care that their products may actually cause breast cancer?

If we refuse to buy any product with a pink ribbon on it, these corporations might think twice about offering them for sale. But, that is easier said than done.

The commercialization of Breast Cancer started many years ago but has accelerated in recent years. Most corporations now have within their marketing departments, executives who are in charge of "Cause Marketing," which is defined as:

A type of marketing involving the cooperative efforts of a for-profit business and a non-profit organization for mutual benefit. Housed in the marketing divisions of corporations, this marketing approach has three primary objectives: (1) to build a reputation as a good corporate citizen, (2) to deepen employee loyalty through employee matching and cause related volunteerism, and (3) to increase sales.

Cause Marketing, as applied to Breast Cancer Awareness Month, has made hundreds of millions, if not billions of dollars for these corporations.

So, our logical question would be, "Where does the money go?" No one seems to know, including me.

I am a longtime member of The Society of Professional Journalists and have won my share of awards in years past as an investigative journalist exposing corruption in local governments and law enforcement cover-ups. I am certainly an experienced investigator.

That said, I still have no idea where the hundreds of millions of dollars in donations and purchased pink ribbon goods actually end up. That should scare everyone, as it does me.

There are far too many companies, organizations, and promotions to track, and very few of them are transparent enough to evaluate. Cause marketing is cast as everything from the saving grace, to the necessarily evil, to the pinkwashing pilferer. There is probably some truth in each characterization. Like everything, there is a context, so let's put it there:

There are more than 1,400 registered nonprofit entities in the United States doing *something* oriented to breast cancer. Billions of dollars have been invested in breast cancer related programs, research, services, and awareness activities over the years.

Of these, more than 300 have no revenues at all; about another 300 have revenues under $50,000; 300 more raise between $100,000 and

$500,000; and some 200 have contributions between $500,000 and $15 million. Susan G. Komen for the Cure, the largest breast cancer charity, received $420 million in revenues in 2011, with $175 million coming from contributions and grants.

In 2021, they have made it more difficult than ever to determine exactly what their true donations number is, with very few even caring if their donation goes where Komen promises it will. This is one reason they only have a Gold Seal of Transparency, instead of the highest Seal, The Platinum Seal, the award that The Becky Baker Foundation has had two years running now.

It appears that Komen's most recent donations are down close to 40% from ten years ago, as many are finally realizing something stinks in this industry and have finally decided to stop throwing away their money.

In total, the nonprofit sector raises an estimated $2.5 to $3.25 billion for breast cancer in any given fiscal year and, between federal funding and the top private foundations, the U.S. spends more than $1 billion annually on breast cancer research.

Although no one knows exactly what this research entails or who does the researching, that number continues to rise each year. Further, no one knows how much is spent on all of those pink ribbon products and fundraising activities that are off the formal grid.

From 1993 to 2004, The Cone Corporate Citizenship Study, christened by the Cone marketing firm, found that about 85 percent of consumers were likely to switch to a new brand of similar price and quality if the new brand were associated with a cause.

The pink ribbon came on the scene in the early 1990s as the symbol for breast cancer awareness, and breast cancer activists had already done the hard work of de-stigmatizing breast cancer.

They increased support programs, funded research, and moved breast cancer into the public limelight. This breast cancer movement had made a real impact on raising awareness of the disease and institutionalizing support. Once breast cancer was out in the open as a good and moral cause, companies lined up to capitalize on the pink ribbon's public appeal. Associating with the mother of all causes, corporations could buoy their public images and their bottom lines.

Cause marketing donations were estimated to reach $1.78 billion in 2013, the most recent year we can find, for a range of causes. This amount pales in comparison to the profits companies bring in from their pink ribbon campaigns. While it is impossible to track exactly how much companies profit, there are a few major examples that show a trend:

Yoplait Yogurt of General Mills
The number one yogurt in America, as popular as Cheerios, Betty Crocker, and Pillsbury, accounts for $1.1 billion of GM's $11.2 billion in sales.

In 1998, Yoplait teamed up with Susan G. Komen For The Cure to create the "Save Lids to Save Lives" campaign. Every October, the company sells yogurt (now without the growth hormone rBGH, thanks to Breast Cancer Action) topped with pink lids. Consumers send the lids to a collection center or log their "redemption codes" through the Yoplait website during a specific time period. Yoplait then donates 10 cents per lid, with a guaranteed minimum donation of $500,000 and cap of $1.5 million.

In 2008, Yoplait consumers redeemed over 15 million pink lids, hitting the cap. The 15 million yogurts less the 10-cents-per-lid donation, yields about $5.9 million in sales. That fiscal year, GM reported a 14 percent sales jump for the Yoplait division.

Ford Mustang Warriors in Pink Emblem

In 2006, *Ford Motor Company* launched the *Warriors in Pink campaign.* The company, in 2008, offered a Ford Mustang with Warriors in Pink package on its Mustang coupe, convertible, and glass roof coupe. The package included a pink ribbon and pony fender badge, pink ribbon rocker tape and hood striping, charcoal leather trimmed seats with pink stitching, and charcoal floor mats with pink ribbon and contrast stitching.

The limited-edition 2008 Mustang with Warriors in Pink package donated $250 per sale to Susan G. Komen for the Cure, totaling over $500,000. Limited to 2,500 units, Ford had to sell 2,000 cars to make the donation.

The special edition was priced from $28,899 to $34,584. The Warriors in Pink package added $1,795 and automatic transmission was required, adding another $1,250. Ford's sales had been down 32 percent in 2008, so expanding the consumer base with this special edition vehicle could help offset the decline.

By December 2009, Ford Mustang sales were up 62 percent, with the Warriors in Pink package accounting for most of that increase.

American Airlines Miles for The Cure

American Airlines expanded its corporate partnership with Komen also in 2008. The airline faced near bankruptcy, with high fuel prices, low consumer demand, debt, and an aging fleet, but entered into a Promise Grant with Komen that was earmarked for the Morgan Welch Inflammatory Breast Cancer Research Program and Clinic.

The partnership would generate $8 million in 8 years through the airline's "Miles for the Cure" program, gift cards, annual celebrity golf and tennis event, and other promotions.

American Airlines would more than cover the $1 million per year allocation. By July 2010, American's performance had already improved "$440 million over the first quarter. The company saw its first operating profit since the third quarter of 2007."

The *National Football League* (NFL)

Pro football started supporting Breast Cancer Awareness Month in 2009 with the "A Crucial Catch" campaign – a nationwide screening reminder to "help women stay healthy." Done in collaboration with the America Cancer Society, the initiative encourages women 40 and older to get annual mammograms. The NFL also sells pink merchandise to raise money for the American Cancer Society.

Business Insider reported that for every $100 in pink merchandise sold $12.50 went to the NFL, of which $11.25 was donated to the

American Cancer Society. The remaining amount was divided between the company that makes the merchandise (37.5 percent) and the company that sells it (50 percent). The manufacturer/seller is often the NFL itself or the individual teams. Again, it is difficult, if not impossible, to track the exact numbers.

The pink ribbon has become a safe bet for corporate investment and, for some, a reliable revenue or profit stream. Nonprofits get some money and free advertising, and companies get to use a social cause to create an image of caring and social responsibility. But is it really benefiting the cause? Ironically, consumers who buy cause marketing products end up giving less money to a social cause or charity, according to a study in the Journal of Consumer Psychology.

Furthermore, as Porter and Kramer argue in the Harvard Business Review, "as long as companies remain focused on the public relations benefit of their contributions instead of impact achieved, they will sacrifice opportunities to create social value. (p. 15)." Social value goes beyond *perceived* good will and dollars donated.

Breast cancer may still be the darling of corporate America, but cause marketing agents should be aware. While consumers seem to like supporting causes with their purchases, Cone Communications also found that they are willing to boycott companies that behave irresponsibly. Exploiting a disease for profit may be one of the most irresponsible (and evil) behaviors of all.

When Komen was outed for donating money to Planned Parenthood for abortions with funds that were donated to them for breast cancer research, their reputation was hammered and remains soiled today. They have lost millions in donations from angry supporters, and continue to do so.

Our voices do matter. Please do not participate in October's Breast Cancer Awareness campaign. Don't buy anything pink. Give your hard-earned money to the foundation of your choice that you know is honoring their word and is completely transparent with all their donations. We have the power to force accountably. Let's rise up and do so.

Section Two

**Preventing Breast Cancer
in Your Loved One**

Chapter Nine
Supporting Your Loved One At All Costs

"Love looks not with the eyes, but with the mind, and therefore is winged Cupid painted blind."
— **William Shakespeare**

In my introduction to this book, I recounted for you the partial story of how I learned that Becky was sick: stubbed her toe on cart at COSTCO; rushed to emergency center; two hours later transferred to cancer ward; oncologist asks to speak to me in hallway; oncologist, with no emotion and in a robotic way, says the following to me:

"Becky has stage IV metastatic ER Positive Breast Cancer. She has three months to live, so get your affairs in order."

Now, I'd like to finish that story, to provide an example of what I mean by "**supporting**" your loved one at all costs. After the chief oncologist told me that Becky was going to die in three months, she wanted to go tell Becky this news so that she could "get her affairs in order."

I told the oncologist three things:

'You are not going to tell Becky that.'
'Becky is not going to die in three months.'
'You are not God, so stop acting like you are.'

She looked stunned. It appeared that she was not used to being confronted or told "no." She shrugged and walked away.

I headed down the hallway to find the coffee pot and when I returned to Becky's suite, the oncologist was at Becky's side telling her she only had three months to live.

Yep. She sure did that after I gave her specific orders not to.

So I kind of lost it. It didn't talk long for the oncologist to threaten me with removal from the hospital if I didn't stop.

So I didn't stop.

She summoned two security guards. I looked at them and told the oncologist that it would take a few more, bigger guards, to get me out. Soon, a few more bigger guards appeared and I was physically removed from the hospital.

Needless to say, Becky was beside herself. She had just been told that her life was going to end, badly, in three months, and then she watched as her husband was forcibly removed from the hospital. She was not happy with me, to be sure.

I was back at the hospital in no time, after speaking with my attorney, and as I entered Becky's suite, her look was one I will never forget. It was one of hopelessness.

She started to tell me that she needed to update her will and I immediately stopped her.

"You're not going to die in three months," I told her.

She said, "You are not the doctor. You are only my husband and know nothing about breast cancer." I told her that while that is true, I know three things:

I know you;
I know you are not going to die in three months; and
I know the oncologist is not God.

Not surprisingly, she did not believe any of my statements.

I knew that I had to convince her and do so fast. I am a positive person and know the importance of a mindset that always sees the best in any situation. Becky was not a positive person, always seeing the glass of water as half empty, never half full. I knew the longer she believed that she would die in three months, the more likely that would be.

So, I fired off a Letter of Intent to sue the hospital and the oncologist. I didn't want money, I only wanted two things:

First, I wanted the hospital to amend their Mission Statement to include a statement that would prohibit any doctor from putting an expiration date on the lives of their patients by telling them they had three months to live.

Second, I wanted the chief oncologist fired. Harsh? Not at all. What was "harsh" was the challenge I now had to convince Becky she would not die in three months, as this oncologist had so boldly claimed. There are times that these doctors, just like our elected officials, need to be reminded that they work for us.

I won on both accounts, although the official word on the chief oncologist was that she left the hospital to "take a position in research in another state."

Becky was beginning to believe she might live past the three months, and four months later when she was still alive, her attitude changed to one of hope. She was ready to fight now and fight she did!

I gave you the rest of the story so you might understand what I mean by supporting your loved one. While I was certainly unconventional (getting thrown out of the hospital) in standing up for my wife, it was what she needed to survive as she lived 37 months beyond those three, and many would not have known she was sick until the last couple months. There was a time, about two years in, when I really believed she was healed. But it was not to be.

Did I overreact to the expiration words of the oncologist? Did I have no right to demand the termination of this doctor?

I leave you with this true story: On Christmas morning, 2017, a full four years after the initial hospital "event," I had a man approach me at a restaurant while I was on the road with my #Race4Prevention Tour. He said that he had followed Becky and the launching of the Foundation after her death on Easter Sunday morning of that year. He had read the media reports about the car, had read my mission, and had read "Becky's Story" on my website. He asked if I had a minute to chat and we sat down together.

He wanted to talk about his wife, who earlier in the year had been diagnosed with stage IV, ER positive metastatic breast cancer, just like Becky.

He told me that once diagnosed, their oncologist told both he and his wife that she had "three months to live so please get your affairs in order." Sound familiar?

Being familiar with my Foundation and Becky, he asked his wife to look at the site with him. They read Becky's Story, where she recounts her desire to fight the disease with her LAFF2LIVE model: Lifestyle, Attitude, Food and Faith. They read together how Becky refused chemo and drugs. How she woke up every morning and said, "I am not going to die today!"

He asked his wife to follow the same path. Her oncologist had already ordered a strict regimen of chemo and drugs, even iBRANCE, the new drug that might extend her life a month or so, to the tune of $250,000 per year without insurance coverage.

After spending hours on the website reading Becky's detailed vision of how to fight this evil disease, he told me that he begged his wife to follow Becky's path, and not the path of the oncologist.

She told him that she just could not. "I am in tears over Becky's story," she told her husband, "but Becky was not a doctor. My doctor is highly acclaimed and if she says I need to do this, I must follow her."

I asked him what happened. He paused, looked up at me with tears running down his face and said, "She died, almost three months to the day of when her doctor told her she would. I don't know how I can go on without her."

The support we give our loved ones may vary and may even seem drastic at the time. It is up to you to determine how far might be too far. Is getting thrown out of the hospital worth it if it shows your wife you are one hundred percent committed to supporting her? That's your decision to make.

I have no doubt that had Becky continued to believe her oncologist, who did not know her, instead of me, who did, she would have died in three months.

Chapter Ten
Becky's LAFF2LIVE Program

by Becky Baker

"Most of the important things in the world have been accomplished by people who have kept on trying when there seemed to be no hope at all."
— **Dale Carnegie**

I have talked much about Becky so far in this book, and I think it is now time for you to hear from her. These are her words that were written about a year and a half after she was diagnosed. The chapter concludes with her final update. Please honor her as you read these words.

IN DECEMBER OF 2013, I WAS DIAGNOSED WITH STAGE IV METASTATIC BREAST CANCER. I WAS GIVEN THREE MONTHS TO LIVE BY THE ONCOLOGISTS AT WAKE FOREST BAPTIST CANCER CENTER IN WINSTON-SALEM, NORTH CAROLINA.

If you're reading this, sadly you too may know that feeling of helplessness that comes over you when you first hear those terrifying words: "You've got cancer."

At first, I thought I was going to die. After all, the expert cancer doctors told me I was. They immediately began talking about "quality of life" for the time I had left — three months.

Their "quality of life" discussion always included pain management, chemotherapy and radiation, with the possibility of surgery.

When one of the most decorated and respected cancer specialists puts a time limit on my remaining days on this earth, who am I to disagree? I'm not the expert, the doctors are. I was in shock and probably at the lowest point in my life.

My husband though, would have none of it. To put it mildly, he went "viral." He demanded that the doctors immediately stop putting a time limit on the days left in my life. I remember well as he raised his voice to the oncologists — over and over again — saying "How dare you tell my wife she is going to die in three months! Who the hell do you think you are, God?"

Why was Rick so convinced that I was not going to die?

Didn't he understand that I was at Stage IV and very few come back from that? Did he not hear the doctors tell us that once the cancer had learned to travel from my breast, it took over my spine and was present in my ribs, sternum, and the head of my femurs?

Was he ignoring the fact that I had compression fractures in my vertebra, three cracked ribs, a fractured sternum and the cancer had weakened my femur necks putting me at great risk of breaking a hip?

Were I to break a hip, my chances for recovery would be slim to none. Did he not even consider the national survival rate statistics for stage four breast cancer patients?

According to the National Cancer Institute's Seer database, in 2013, there were close to 250,000 new breast cancer cases, with over 40,000 deaths in the U.S. alone. Most of those cases were localized, meaning they were confined to the primary site, the breast for example. The five-year survival rate for localized breast cancer, or stages one and two, is over 98 percent. But I had Stage IV, and the five-year survival rate for my advanced stage and type of cancer is less than five percent.

Still, Rick kept telling me I was not going to die, regardless of what the doctors said, and you know what? I began to believe him.

I agreed to the 10 radiation treatments the doctors recommended immediately after my diagnosis. These treatments targeted my right femur neck, which was the most involved, and compression fractures in my back. They told me it was mandatory to stabilize the areas worst hit. When I had completed radiation, they told me I needed to begin a regimen of chemotherapy, a monthly injection to help rebuild my bones, and, possibly, additional radiation.

I was wheeled, that's right, in a wheelchair, to the pod where I received my first bone building injection. This was also the area where chemotherapy is administered. It was decorated in soothing colors and looked brand new. The nurses were very nice and supportive.

But, what struck me most were the looks on the faces of the other patients. For the most part they looked worn out, and many looked lost in hopelessness. Those who made eye contact with me expressed sorrow and pity that I was about to join their ranks.

That did it. I knew right then that chemotherapy was not right for me. If I only had three months to live, I was not going to live it like this. Normally, as anyone who knows me will attest, I respect authority almost to a fault. If an authority figure tells me that I have to do something, I do it. Once I made my decision though, I immediately felt at peace with it.

So, Rick and I both became obsessed with researching other treatments to fight, and beat, this evil disease.

We found that there were countless treatments, supplements, and protocols available, all claiming to "heal, cure, or prevent cancer." If you've done any kind of online search, you know what I'm talking about. I'm not here to recommend or condemn any of them, although there is a list of some of the sites we utilized and you can feel free to contact us for that information.

After narrowing the options down to a more manageable size, we came up with our own course of action to beat this beast of a disease.

Now, please understand, I am not a doctor. I would never recommend that you ignore the advice of your oncologist. We chose to try a more natural healing path over the past 20 months, and it appears to be working for me. This path I am now committed to hasn't just given me an additional 17 months from the doctor's original diagnosis, it has "stabilized my cancer," according to my oncologist.

While other doctors might claim I am in "remission," my doctor doesn't like to use that word. I will never be "cancer free," but I believe that I can live to old age by continuing the path I am now on. The cancer will not conquer me or end my life.

Not that long ago, I needed a walker to move around the house and a grabber to pick up my socks from the floor. I couldn't drive. I couldn't go up or down stairs.

I couldn't cook or clean or play with the dogs. I couldn't do any of the basic things we take for granted every day. Thankfully, I had the help and support of my wonderful husband, Rick. He did everything for me, including being my chief advocate, an absolute necessity for anyone with a health issue.

In short, today I no longer even know where my walker is. I actually walk distances for exercise now. I still have to be mindful of my limitations, but have started physical therapy to increase my strength and range of motion. But, the best part for me is that I have plants! This Spring, I planted more flowers, vegetables, and herbs than any one person should.

It just felt so good to once again get my hands in the dirt and be able to create beautiful designs with plant material, that I went a little crazy. Ok, quite a bit crazy. Everything is planted in containers so that it's easier for me to help maintain them, and I still need some help from Rick, but I don't care. I get to play in the dirt!

My purpose here is to encourage all breast cancer patients and, maybe more importantly, those who have not heard those terrible words: "You've got cancer." The changes we've made in our lives aren't earth shattering. They're just things that made sense to us as we moved forward in our battle for wellness. We believe that everyone can benefit from these changes. And the best thing is, you have nothing to lose by trying it.

If I can help encourage you in any way, I would love to talk to you!

So, what exactly is the path we've chosen for my fight against breast cancer? To keep it simple we've condensed it to these four things: *Lifestyle, Attitude, Food and Faith.*

Here is a summary of each piece of the LAFF path:

Lifestyle

We have done an overall assessment of what emotions and triggers could have played a role in cancer setting up camp in my body. Lifestyle is sort of a catchall for things you do in your everyday life that can have a detrimental effect on your well-being.

Number one on the hit parade is stress. Everyone has stress. It's a fact of life. But, we can all do little things to alleviate the level of stress our minds and bodies have to deal with on a daily basis. It will take some conscious effort on your part, but it can be done.

The other part of the stress equation, is how you react to it. Do you get even more stressed just thinking about how much stress you're under?

This is a vicious cycle that many of us find ourselves in. We even become stressed when we think there isn't enough stress, assuming that something must be wrong. How out of whack is that?

Worry is another energy sink. We waste so much of the present time worrying about what may or may not happen in the future. The same can be said for wasting our energy worrying about the past. If you're letting the past or the future monopolize your thoughts, you're not really living in the present, and you're certainly not enjoying it.

As simple as it sounds, a good night's sleep is vital for a healthy mind and body. I know that this is easier said than done, but it's another one of those things that we became more aware of and made a concerted effort to work on.

Physical activity helps with a lot of the other things in the lifestyle category. It's a great stress reliever, it helps you sleep if you've had a good workout earlier in the day, and it helps keep the many systems of your body working in tiptop form. The alternative lack of activity can lead to many physical problems, plus, you won't get the kick of endorphins to brighten your mood.

We will expand on all of these and offer suggestions later but let me just state right now that there is one little word that you will need to use more regularly. You will need to learn to say (and mean) no!

Attitude

Having a positive attitude is so important in everything you do and is huge in the healing process. I don't mean being so overly positive that you become delusional about the fact that you are ill. The old "if I ignore it and say I'm fine, it'll go away" tactic doesn't usually work in real life. It didn't for me anyway…

Rather, don't dwell on the illness, or whatever your problem may be, and ignore all the good things that may be happening in your life. I've always been an upbeat person, so maybe this one was easier for me than it may be for you. I just never let myself wallow in self-pity or let my disease define me.

I appreciate even the little things more now than I ever have. I enjoy my time with family and friends. I appreciate the antics of our four furry kids. I plant and nurture beautiful flowers just because I can. It doesn't matter if anyone else sees them. The bees, the butterflies, and I enjoy them to their fullest.

Food

What we put in our mouths has probably been the biggest change for Rick and me. We will get into the particulars later, but suffice it to say, that when we started analyzing what we consumed in the name of nutrition, we were appalled.

We switched to a diet that consists of organic whenever possible, much less animal protein, little added sugar, less processed/packaged foods, and no Diet Coke. That last one was a biggie for me. My first thought when I was admitted to the hospital was that Rick would have to bring me one in the morning or I wouldn't be able to get through the day. Pretty sad, huh?

Faith

The first thing we did when we heard those terrifying words: "You've got cancer," was pray. We needed God to lay His healing touch on me and we needed His guidance.

We also asked for prayers from family, friends, and the tens of thousands of followers Rick had acquired over the years from his writing. We had, and still have, thousands of wonderful people lifting us up in prayer every day.

We felt a sense of peace knowing that we were covered by His grace. Although we didn't know what the future would hold, or even how much of a future I had, we knew that God was in charge and everything would be okay.

Without this faith we may have bought into the prediction of the doctors who said I only three months to live. We knew that only God knows when we will breathe our last on this earth, and although doctors have lots of knowledge, this sort of proclamation was above their pay grade. But I knew and believed.

Becky's Final Update, December, 2016:

I wrote the preceding chapter about a year and a half after I was diagnosed with stage IV breast cancer for my website, LAFF2LIVE.org. So, what has happened in the past year and a half? Well, the cancer is no longer stable or in remission as Rick and I both thought it was. I am a bit weaker from a low hemo count, and I can feel the cancer starting to take over my body, but I am still here! Yes, the cancer is beginning to take its toll, but I have not given up my fight and never will! I will keep fighting! I will not die today! I love you all! Becky.

Rick Update, Easter Sunday, 2017:

Four months after Becky penned this update, and 37 months after she was given just three months to live, Becky passed to her Heavenly home on Easter Sunday morning at 4:58 a.m. The doctors at Wake Forest Baptist Hospital, who originally thought she was delusional for believing she could live longer than three months, have often used Becky as a case study in how organic food, positive attitude, and prayer may indeed extend the life of a terminally-ill breast cancer patient who refuses chemo or drugs.

But in the end, the cancer won and a breast cancer death is one of the most horrific deaths for the patient and the loved ones who are left behind. Before Becky was diagnosed, she was close to six feet tall and weighed 130 pounds. At her passing, she was 5'8 and barely 60 pounds. Some of her own family members would not go see her in those final days because they didn't want to "remember her that way."

In those final minutes that I had with her, I doubt she was aware that I was holding her hand and kissing her forehead. Then, suddenly, I watched her smile, as she took her last labored breath on this earth. No more pain. No more physical body to weigh down her soul. Only joy for her now. Her journey was complete and my loss was Heaven's gain.

A few weeks before Becky passed away, we were having a conversation about the future. As she looked out our kitchen window, watching the dogs run and play on the property, she looked at me and said, "I'm just sorry that no one will ever remember my name." I was stunned and had to hold back the tears.

After I regained my composure, I promised her that 'no one would ever forget her name.' So, three weeks after she passed away, I launched The Becky Baker Foundation. An IRS nonprofit 501(C)(3) charity organization that would be committed to providing thousands of free mammograms and thermograms to women (and men) who could not afford the screening. To date, the FDN has provided over 2,400 free mammograms and thermograms for the underinsured and uninsured.

Chapter Eleven
Design Your Own Proactive Plan

"Never let anyone define you. You are the only person who defines you. No one can speak for you. Only you speak for you. You are your only voice."
— **Terry Crews**

A breast cancer death, as with any death, is tragic. However, a breast cancer death is something that the surviving family members will never forget.

I described for you earlier what happened to Becky's body when that tumor the size of a BB metastasized and spread throughout her bones. Here's a bit more detail: She had four compression fractures on her vertebrae, three fractured ribs, a fractured sternum, and both hip femurs were in danger of splintering. If she were to turn around too quickly, she would break her hip. We were watching TV one night and she had a hard sneeze. That sneeze fractured another rib.

This was a woman who just a short time earlier was almost six feet tall, in perfect health, had hiked many 14ers in Colorado, and was the Master "Bird Lady" at the Phoenix Zoo, where birds of prey from Condors to Falcons would coo on her shoulder and give her beak kisses.

Now, her body was disintegrating, eaten up by breast cancer, a disease that has a mind of its own and is not understood or conquered by even the greatest of human geniuses.

As I have mentioned throughout this book, it is my prayer that you read and take to your soul every word printed here so that you and your loved one will hopefully never go through what Becky and I did.

Again, had Becky taken care of that minute lump in her left breast once she discovered it, she would most likely still be here today. Much of what I write here is to encourage you to do whatever it takes to not get to this place of despair.

This chapter is designed for those who have no breast cancer in their lives. The following chapters are for those families that have heard those three fateful words: "You've Got Cancer."

You are living the dream, and probably never even considered those words being directed to your wife or girlfriend, until you started reading this book! Everyone else gets breast cancer, but not your loved one, even though you now know that close to one-in-seven women in the U.S. will be diagnosed with breast cancer in their lifetimes.

Those are high odds and hopefully will motivate you to start your plan for breast cancer prevention today and not wait. But just in case you need more motivation, here it is:

I have mentioned that I thought Becky had been healed at about the two-and-a-half-year mark. She looked just like you and me. While a bit slower, and she tired easily, she had been off her walker so long neither one of us knew where it was.

It was Christmas, 2016, when her condition began to change. She told me her stomach would ache now for no reason at all. Back to the doc we went, and the news was a blow: The pain was breast cancer related, which had possibly returned with a vengeance. Or, maybe not "returned" because it had never gone away, just put to sleep because Becky had stopped feeding it as she had been committed to only organic, healthy foods since her diagnosis in December of 2013.

However, her breast cancer had awakened and now with an energy we had not seen. Once I learned what was to follow, I wasn't sure I was strong enough to cope.

I had been her rock for three years, never wavering; I had stood up to a world-renowned oncologist, getting tossed from the hospital in the process; threatened to sue one of the largest hospitals in the state if my demands were not met, which they were; encouraged Becky to stand tall when other doctors accused her of being "irresponsible with her body" when she refused chemo; begged her to write her story so that she could help the thousands of others in her same stage, and she has; and told her every day that she would not die on that day!

But this new turn of events, I just wasn't sure I could handle.

In January, a month after Becky first complained of mid-section pain, her stomach began to grow. Larger and larger, and so off to the doc again.

We were told that this was fluid, as a direct result of her breast cancer and the destruction it was causing all her organs now. The doc said she needed to come back to the hospital weekly going forward to be "drained." Yep, drained.

They set us up for the next day. When we arrived, Becky was laid on the table, her mid-section exposed where they inserted a port for the draining.

After all I had been through, this was the hardest for me to watch. The tubes were hooked up, and she began to "drain." One liter, two, three, four, five, six. Six liters and her belly was finally drained. She no longer looked to be nine months pregnant after a gallon and a half of that nasty fluid had been sucked from her body. She was now in great pain because all those organs that had been compressed and pushed aside by the fluid were now free to move back into place. Becky said that pain was worse than the pressure of all that fluid in her body.

We would return to that hospital bed every week through mid-February, when we were told Becky needed to be drained twice a week.

This was so hard on Becky that I asked if I could be certified to do this at home, in our bed. The medical staff agreed and taught me what and how to do something that I never thought I had the strength to do.

I was sent home with a case of highly sterile one-liter bags, a number of tubes, clips, and a special smock to wear when draining her. It was a very real possibility that Becky could get infected now that she was in a non-sterile environment such as our bed when the draining took place. That could certainly kill her.

The next couple weeks of February were especially hard on both of us. I was not an expert at this yet and made mistakes. Once, I didn't "click" the hose correctly, and her fluid leaked all over her and the bed. Do I need to tell you how it smelled? Or the clean-up process? Good, I won't.

I became an expert at this though by the first week of March. Twice a week through mid-March, then as that evil fluid refilled her midsection more quickly now, three, then four, then five times a week.

By the first week of April, I was draining her every day and still losing ground. Five to six liters of fluid, a gallon and a half, every day. Her pain was so intense now, as her body never had a chance to recover from the drain the day before.

Then, the saddest day of my life, and hers, came to be. Becky Baker, the woman who hiked all those 14ers; the woman who had spent the past three years plus courageously fighting this evil disease, who once was the perfect example of health, said this to me:

"Rick, please take me to Hospice."

I will never forget as they put her on that stretcher in our bedroom and wheeled her out to the awaiting ambulance. Our three dogs: Penny, our Great White Pyrenees; Charlie, our Pyrenees/Husky; and Hoover, our English Cream Golden, watched and seemed so confused and even sad. They sat on the porch and watched as the ambulance slowly drove down our 400-foot drive and then she was gone.

Three days later, Becky asked me to bring Charlie to see her at hospice. As we entered her room, and she called him over, he didn't know who she was. He didn't recognize her. Her favorite of all our kiddos didn't know who she was. The sadness of this fact was written all over Becky's face.

In fact, Becky's physical appearance had deteriorated so quickly, she almost looked subhuman. Even some of her own family members refused to go and visit her the last week of her life. They said that they could not handle "remembering her that way." Their loss.

Becky would live only two more weeks. She would be drained every day and the last week or so, she ate nothing and existed only on morphine, the pain so unbearable. She passed away at 4:58 a.m. on Easter Sunday morning, April 16, 2017.

An hour after she left this planet, I was still numb and in a daze. I knew this day would come but was surprisingly not ready for it. After I said my final goodbyes to her, and kissed her still-warm face, they came to take her away. I needed to run home quickly to feed our dogs, as I had been at her bedside for 12 hours straight. As I started the car, the radio was on and this song by Mercy Me started to play as I began to drive:

They say sometimes you win some
Sometimes you lose some
And right now, right now I'm losing bad
I've stood on this stage night after night
Reminding the broken it'll be alright
But right now, oh right now I just can't

*It's easy to sing
When there's nothing to bring me down
But what will I say
When I'm held to the flame
Like I am right now*

*I know You're able and I know You can
Save through the fire with Your mighty hand
But even if You don't
My hope is You alone*

*They say it only takes a little faith
To move a mountain
Good thing
A little faith is all I have right now
But God, when You choose
To leave mountains unmovable
Give me the strength to be able to sing
It is well with my soul*

*I know You're able and I know You can
Save through the fire with Your mighty hand
But even if You don't
My hope is You alone
I know the sorrow, and I know the hurt
Would all go away if You'd just say the word
But even if You don't
My hope is You alone*

*You've been faithful, You've been good
All of my days
Jesus, I will cling to You*

Come what may
'Cause I know You're able
I know You can

I know You're able and I know You can
Save through the fire with Your mighty hand
But even if You don't
My hope is You alone
I know the sorrow, and I know the hurt
Would all go away if You'd just say the word
But even if You don't
My hope is You alone

My hope is you alone

It is well with my soul
It is well, it is well with my soul

(By Crystal Lewis, Tim Timmons, Ben Glover, February 17, 2017. With permission)

But it wasn't well with my soul, and some days even now, it is still not. Why didn't I see she was sick? What could I have done differently that might have saved her? Was I strong enough? Was I the reason she got sick because I wasn't a good enough husband? The questions still come, even today, almost four years later.

Was this story about draining Becky too morbid for you? Do you think you could do what I did? Maybe yes, but I know husbands who have walked away too. If you don't want to find out, then start today with your commitment to preventing breast cancer in your loved ones.

Remember, only about five percent of those diagnosed with breast cancer annually are genetic or hereditary. Breast cancer can be preventable. You must know what to look for and always be on the alert.

Chapter Twelve
Knowing Breast Cancer Stages

There's no such thing as a bad decision,
just bad information.
—**Unknown**

Even if you know little about breast cancer, you probably know that stage IV of any cancer is the worst and deadliest of the stages. The odds are not great that a stage IV breast cancer patient will fully recover and often times this stage is fatal.

But, what about the other stages? What are they and how does the medical field determine which stage you are?

Simply put, the stage of a breast cancer is determined by the cancer's characteristics, such as how large it is and whether or not it is non-invasive, meaning has it remained within its original location, or has become invasive, having spread outside the breast to other parts of the body.

So, stage 0 means the cancer is still limited to the breast and stages I, II, III, and IV describe how the cancer has left the breast and where it has traveled in the body, as well as the extent of the damage.

When Becky first discovered that small lump in her left breast in March of 2013, it was the size of a BB, and she was at stage 0. Had she immediately been checked out, the worst-case scenario most likely would have been a mastectomy. But she didn't get it checked out.

So, that small tumor began to grow and it apparently grew quickly, although it may have been present in her breast for years. I will address that later in this chapter.

She went from stage 0 to stage 1 in probably a month or two. The tumor now began to grow. No longer limited to that one area of her breast, it began to spread throughout the healthy tissue of her breast and into other parts of her body, looking for other healthy tissue and organs to consume. It attacked her underarm lymph nodes and then went for her vertebrae.

Now, two months removed from finding the small lump, her breast cancer was most likely at stage II and traveling aggressively. Possibly fueled by her love of Diet Coke, or maybe it was her daily stress of events that occurred many years earlier in her life that she had never resolved. Either way, the cancer was now turbo-charged.

By July or so, her cancer had metastasized and was now taking over her ribs and more vertebrae. She had arrived at stage III.

By October, the cancer had spread to her femur necks, weakening her hip joints which were now in danger of breaking, and had begun to travel up her spine, to her rib cage, and had weakened her sternum enough that it cracked on its own. Two months later, she stubbed her toe at COSTCO, and was officially placed at stage IV.

To backtrack a bit, I mentioned earlier in this chapter that Becky may have had that small tumor in her left breast prior to when she discovered it. I say this because of that slight deformity in her breast that I saw on our wedding night. As I found out later, her breast had begun to deform in that area a year or so earlier.

A couple of days before she passed away, the nurse came in to change her gown and so I helped move Becky to do this. I will never forget what I saw when her gown was removed: Most of her left breast was gone, eaten away by the cancer, leaving a gaping, deep open wound, right where she had originally discovered the small lump. Was that lump present yet dormant years before she discovered it? It is possible.

Officially, the breast cancer staging system is called the TNM system and it is overseen by the American Joint Committee on Cancer (AJCC). The AJCC is a group of cancer experts who oversee how cancer is classified and communicated. This is to ensure that all doctors and treatment facilities are describing cancer in a uniform way so that the treatment results of all people can be compared and understood.

Up until 2018, the stage number was calculated based on just three clinical characteristics, T, N, and M:

• *the size of the cancer tumor and whether or not it has grown into nearby tissue (T)*

• *whether cancer is in the lymph nodes (N)*

• *whether the cancer has spread to other parts of the body beyond the breast (M)*

Numbers or letters after T, N, and M give more details about each characteristic. Higher numbers mean the cancer is more advanced. In 2018, the AJCC added information about tumor grade, hormone-receptor status, HER2 status and Oncotype DX test results that have made determining the stage of a breast cancer more complex, but also more accurate.

Here's my attempt at a simple definition of each stage:

Stage 0
This stage describes non-invasive breast cancers. In stage 0, there is no evidence of cancer cells or non-cancerous abnormal cells breaking out of the part of the breast in which they started or getting through to or invading neighboring normal tissue.

Stage I
Stage I describes invasive breast cancer (cancer cells are breaking through to or invading normal surrounding breast tissue). Stage I is divided into subcategories known as IA and IB. (You can search the Internet to learn more about these subcategories.)

Stage II
Stage II is also divided into subcategories known as IIA and IIB. In general, stage IIA describes invasive breast cancer in which: no tumor can be found in the breast, but cancer (larger than 2 millimeters [mm]) is

found in 1 to 3 axillary lymph nodes (the lymph nodes under the arm) or in the lymph nodes near the breast bone (found during a sentinel node biopsy) or; the tumor measures 2 centimeters (cm) or smaller and has spread to the axillary lymph nodes or; the tumor is larger than 2 cm but not larger than 5 cm and has not spread to the axillary lymph nodes.

Stage III

Stage III is divided into three subcategories known as IIIA, IIIB, and IIIC. In general, stage IIIA describes invasive breast cancer in which either: no tumor is found in the breast or the tumor may be any size; cancer is found in 4 to 9 axillary lymph nodes or in the lymph nodes near the breastbone or; the tumor is larger than 5 centimeters (cm); small groups of breast cancer cells (larger than 0.2 millimeter [mm] but not larger than 2 mm) are found in the lymph nodes or; the tumor is larger than 5 cm; cancer has spread to 1 to 3 axillary lymph nodes or to the lymph nodes near the breastbone (found during a sentinel lymph node biopsy).

Stage IV

Stage IV describes invasive breast cancer that has spread beyond the breast and nearby lymph nodes to other organs of the body, such as the lungs, distant lymph nodes, skin, bones, liver, or brain. You may hear the words "advanced" and "metastatic" used to describe stage IV breast cancer. Cancer may be stage IV at first diagnosis, called "de novo" by doctors, or it can be a recurrence of a previous breast cancer that has spread to other parts of the body.

Chapter Thirteen
The Oncologist Plays God

"I find medicine is the best of all trades, because whether you do any good or not, you still get your money."
— **Moliere 1664**

Full disclosure here: I do not really care for oncologists. You probably already know that based on my experience with the Wake Forest Baptist Hospital former Head of Oncology. You know, the one who told Becky she was going to "die in three months" after I explicitly told her not to. She believed her "expert opinion" trumped my wishes as Becky's husband. I only wish this doctor could have seen Becky a full three years after her unconscionable diagnosis. But, shortly after giving Becky her expiration orders, the doctor was given her marching orders, and that was that.

I promise to be as objective as possible and I ask you to read this chapter with an open mind and make no judgements until you have researched on your own the information that I present here.

Let me start by stating my purpose in writing this chapter. That way, you'll know why I have included this subject in the book. Whether your loved one is currently under the care of an oncologist, or God forbid, one day may be.

Here it is: Oncologists are not God, and as such, are not to be blindly or ignorantly believed in any of their recommendations for treatment, longevity of life with the disease, or other opinions pertaining your diagnosis.

Notice, I said not 'blindly believed.' I am not condemning all oncologists, just alerting you to the fact that they are human and every oncologist has one big challenge to overcome, one that many have not:

Their conflict of interest.

Don't listen to me. Read what Dr. Eisenberg, the Medical Director at Marin Cancer Care in Greenbrae, CA, says about this conflict of interest:

"The reason oncologists have been able to grow a practice as large as ours and provide the level of service we do is because of the revenue we obtain from selling chemotherapy drugs and services...

"We are paid more for administering the drugs than we were in the past, so it makes economic sense to administer them more often. Not every doctor is willing to do that. The practices that show some restraint and don't treat everyone who walks through the door with chemo are the ones that are suffering...

"When doctors are paid to "do more" there is always the potential for conflict of interest. Keep in mind that physicians are human beings with the same kinds of responses to financial incentives as everyone

else. Despite our training and promise to put our patient's interest first, we succumb to incentives that often come in the form of more revenue."

Did you read that carefully? Did it scare the bejeebers out of you? Did it shake your trust in these doctors? It should have. Dr. Eisenberg told the truth and in doing so, has shaken the very foundation of Oncology.

Dr. Eisenberg's shocking admission that many oncologists develop a treatment plan for their patients based on how much money they can make is supported by countless examples across the country.

One of the most famous was Dr. Farid Fata, who was sentenced to 45 years in prison in 2015. His second appeal was just denied late last year. Dr. Fata was truly loved by all his breast cancer patients who were under his care. I mean, he was loved. So, what did he do to get almost half a century behind bars?

He told hundreds of his patients that they had breast cancer, even though they didn't. He ordered chemotherapy to people who didn't need it, most of whom didn't have breast cancer at all, and raked it in to the tune of $35 million. Yep, that's a thirty-five with six zeros!

Dr. Fata was convicted of preying on his patients to pad his pockets. The charges against him were shocking: "deliberate misdiagnosis of patients as having cancer," and giving "unnecessary chemotherapy" including to "end-of-life patients who will not benefit."

There are a plethora of studies online that confirm that oncologists are some of the highest paid doctors, with their average income increasing faster than any other specialist in the medical field, but here is the real kicker: More than half their income comes from selling and administering chemotherapy.

Yes, you read that right. Oncologists make a huge profit and as much as two-thirds of their income, in some cases, comes from chemotherapy drugs.

Before Becky got sick, I had this image of doctors as these professionals working selflessly to save the lives of dying people; and most are. But oncologists are human, and as such, many begin to place their ultimate value on money and not the life they are supposed to save.

Their business model is very different from other doctors because you can't buy chemotherapy drugs at your local pharmacy.

Oncologists buy these drugs direct at wholesale prices, then they mark them up and bill the insurance companies or the patient if uninsured. This legal profiting on drugs by doctors is unique to the cancer treatment world. They're making money off the drugs that they demand you take to save your life.

Can we say, "Conflict of Interest?" They're selling you the drugs and charging you for the privilege of putting them in your body. No other doctor can do that.

I have talked to many oncologists who feel "trapped in this system." This billion-dollar cancer treatment industry is controlled by the pharmaceutical companies, who will be the subject of my next book, out later this year.

I know an oncologist in the Eastern U.S. who has turned to the dark side and now places more value on the U.S. dollar than human life. As she once told me, "These patients are going to die anyway no matter what I do, so why not make a buck?" Here's how it works for her:

On any given month, she has close to 100 chemo patients that she has diagnosed with stage III or IV breast cancer. Some have been given the "you have three months to live" expiration date just as Becky was given.

They come in once a month for the chemo drip that lasts four to five hours. They sit in their La-Z-Boy recliners, listening to music or reading their book (which I hope is this one!).

I do not know if any of these patients have been misdiagnosed or are getting unnecessary chemotherapy. Here's what I do know: She is making millions.

Here's how it works:

She sells the chemo to the patient for *about* $4,000 (I use *about* because the drug cocktail may be different in each patient) but buys each treatment wholesale for about $1,800.

Let's do the math: 100 chemo drip patients once a month pay about $4,000 retail for the five-hour IV drip that this oncologist buys wholesale for about $1,800.

This is a net profit of about $2,200 per patient, times the 100 patients is about $220,000 per month, or about $2,640,000 per year.

According to the American Society of Clinical Oncology (ASCO), there are about 10,500 practicing oncologists in the U.S. Certainly, most are ethical and caring doctors who certainly put their patients above making a buck.

However, every single oncologist is faced with the same conflict of interest with their patients. How can you be sure that your doctor places you above the dollar?

One simple question should do it:

"Do you make any commission on the drugs you prescribe me, including buying wholesale, and selling to me at retail?"

That should do it. Any oncologist who accepts a commission for prescribing any chemo drug should not be trusted, in my opinion.

Becky's second oncologist recommended that Becky begin taking IBRANCE, which was a new drug at the time that had been rushed through trials and had no real clinical studies. This drug would cost upwards of a quarter-of-a-million dollars per year for the uninsured. I asked her the above question. She seemed stunned that I would challenge her, but to her credit, after trying to deflect, did admit that she made "a small commission."

Becky then asked her three questions:

1. "Will this drug cure my cancer?"
2. "Will this drug save my life?"
3. "Will I lose my hair, be bedridden, and lay in my own vomit if I take this drug which may extend my life only a month or two?"

Her answer to number one was, "No." Number two was, "No." And, her answer to Becky's third question was, "Yes, most likely."

Our oncologist was not aware I was loaded for bear, having already extensively researched IBRANCE and discussed this treatment with Becky. We probably knew more about the new drug than our doctor did.

I asked her how she could take any commission (especially from a drug that did not have a clear track record of success) and how was this not a conflict of interest. She had no answer.

This is why Becky's first oncologist prescribed many drugs for her upon the initial diagnosis that had nothing to do with her breast cancer. These worthless prescriptions were what first alerted me to the industry marriage of big pharma and oncology. Why did she do it? She was paid a commission by the drug company for every prescription. I was disgusted then, but in the past three years, my disgust has turned to anger and rage. My personal belief is that there is a special place in hell for any doctor who profits financially at the expense of the life they are entrusted to save.

In closing, I encourage you to not be fooled by their appearance or all the degrees that follow their name. If you do not have an instant connection with your oncologist, (this goes for all doctors) if they appear arrogant or hard to communicate with, it may be very hard for you to think straight. If you don't think straight, you are in real danger of making bad decisions. And, bad decisions could cost you your life.

Find another oncologist. If you cannot, contact my Foundation today and we will help find one for you.

Epilogue
Never Give Up

Personally, I have no idea how a breast cancer patient feels. Having supported Becky for those three plus years gave me tremendous, yet at times horrifying, insight to what it must feel like. But, I was never the one fighting or dying from the disease, so I have no idea how she felt deep inside, in her bones and/or her soul.

I know that we are all going to die one day. For me, I hope it is fast and not too painful because I am weak.

Becky was not weak, and as you have learned, her death was slow and very painful. While there were days she wanted to give up, she never did. I want to be more like her.

I have recounted for you in these preceding thirteen chapters some very private events and experiences that I had with Becky. Some very morbid, others very emotional. Most of her family members didn't know much of this until they read this book.

Why do this? Because I do not want you or your loved one to ever have to endure what Becky did. Have I tried to "scare" you into making a commitment to know more about this disease and how it can impact your family? Yep, I sure have. God forbid breast cancer ever visits you or your loved ones but if it does, I want you to be the educated, unwavering rock of support for your loved one, protecting her with your life. And yes, there may be things you are forced to do that you don't think you have the strength to accomplish. But you will surprise yourself and do it for love.

Because "love" is all that really matters on this planet. Not money, not fame, not power. Just love.

In Becky's passing, she has saved hundreds of other women, and quite a few men:

A male Army Colonel, who gave me his Challenge Coin so that I would never forget him; a pro golfer; a mother of five; a famous actress; a newspaper reporter, and a long-haul truck driver.

She saved a 29-year-old young woman; a 40-year-old Uber driver who told me he had many lumps on both breasts and no money for a mammogram. The foundation that bears her name paid for both a mammogram and a thermogram for this man, who is going to make it.

She saved the grandmother from Kansas City; the fashion model from New York City; the waitress from Winston-Salem; the Navajo jewelry maker from Arizona; and the hotel desk clerk who came upon a foundation pen and called for a free screening, just in time as it turned out.

Becky was there for the magazine publisher who read her story, took it to heart, and scheduled a screening that saved her life.

And for the sheriff's deputy, who worked so many hours that she didn't have time to get her screening, until she was forced to.

In her passing, Becky has saved hundreds and provided over 2,400 free screenings for those who are uninsured or underinsured. She has also provided breast cancer prevention education to hundreds of others who in turn scheduled their screening as a result of our foundation's president, Dr. Barb Hughson and her commitment to honoring Becky and to preventing breast cancer.

I will never know how many people Becky has saved or what impact her name and story will have in the future. I only know that I will continue to honor my words to her shortly before she passed away: "*I promise you, Becky Baker, that no one will ever forget your name.*"

Stay alert. Always love. Never give up.